TRIUMPH
OVER TRAUMA

Empowering Sites.com

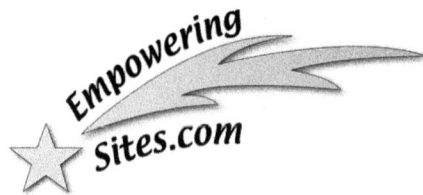

Disclaimer: This book does not replace the advice of a medical professional. Consult your physician before deciding on whether psychedelic medicines can help you.

Edited by Jenny Hansen
Designed by Michelle Fairbanks

TRIUMPH
OVER TRAUMA

**PSYCHEDELIC MEDICINES ARE HELPING
PEOPLE HEAL THEIR TRAUMA,
CHANGE THEIR LIVES,
AND GROW THEIR SPIRITUALITY**

*TRANSFORMATIVE STORIES
TO GUIDE YOU AS YOU EMBARK ON YOUR
OWN HEALING JOURNEY*

RANDALL S. HANSEN, PH.D.

DEDICATION

This book is dedicated to all the people who have healed and been transformed through the use of psychedelic medicines – and all those who will receive the healing and help they need.

TABLE OF CONTENTS

PART THREE: MICRODOSING

PART FOUR: WRAP UP

" "   **INSPIRING QUOTE**
"Trauma is hell on earth. Trauma resolved is a gift
from the gods." – PETER A. LEVINE   **" "**

AUTHOR'S NOTE

It was my distinct privilege – perhaps the biggest of my personal and professional life – to gather the stories and narratives composing most of this book.

Each story is real, all told directly to me via written text or video recordings. There are no composites or fictional characters. Each person's story in this book details their accounts of living their lives, searching for healing and transformation, and partaking in medicines that are still currently illegal at the Federal level – not just in the U.S., but in most of the world.

The stories have been edited only for clarity and style. Where only a first name is listed, it may or may not be a pseudonym, but the author is protecting some elements of their lives. Others are now working in the psychedelics space and share their full names and their websites.

I didn't set out to write a book on psychedelics. In fact, as of about three years ago, I was completely unaware of the healing potential that psychedelics can offer to many people suffering needlessly… hopelessly. Since that time, I have become immersed in this very exciting field of healing and am now ready to share this knowledge – for your healing, your spiritual growth, and your transformation.

Interestingly, the concept for this book came to me during an LSD journey. I was given the entire premise and outline for the book – and shown how important a learning tool this book can be for the many who were like me – unaware of psychedelics but interested in health and wellness… and living one's best life.

My hope is that this book serves as an entry point for you – to discover the enormous potential of these psychedelic plants and medicines for our mental health – and for improving our collective mental health.

Without further ado, I welcome you to my introductory chapters covering all the basics you need to know about psychedelics – and then the truly amazing and powerful stories from people whose lives have been transformed through intentional use of psychedelic medicines.

Finally, this book is for you if you or someone you love is seeking healing, wellness, transformation. This book is for you if you are...

- *interested in learning about the true history of psychedelics for healing.*
- *uncertain about the use and safety of psychedelic medicines.*
- *curious about how one or more of these medicines might change your life.*
- *pursuing major healing and change in your life.*
- *searching for a deeper connection to the mystical, spiritual, and/or the Divine.*
- *wanting more information about how to use a psychedelic medicine safely and effectively.*
- *best convinced by hearing/reading people's stories of healing with these medicines.*

" INSPIRING QUOTE "With psychedelics, if you're fortunate and break through, you understand what is truly of value in life. Material, power, dominance, and territory have no value. People wouldn't fight wars, and the whole system we have currently would fall apart. People would become peaceful, loving citizens, not robots marching around in the dark with all their lights off." – GARY FISHER **"**

INTRODUCTION

We are a people in crisis.
We are in a mental health crisis.
We are in a suicide crisis.
We are in an addiction crisis.
We are in a spiritual crisis.
We are in a wellness crisis.
We are in an abuse crisis.
We are in a pill-popping crisis.

We are in a HEALING crisis.

Not to sound overly dramatic, but we as a society are the unhappiest we have ever been. We all have hidden fears, anxieties, traumas, hurts – and pain, guilt, shame, and anger that are not so hidden. So many of us are broken on the inside… and many of us don't even know it, but all the signs are there.

We are hurting as a community. We are hurting as individuals – and we need healing. These traumas often lead to negative behaviors and consequences. What's worse, we are facing a massive mental health crisis that's been building for decades and is close to a tipping point.

Not only do we have our own traumas to deal with – and by the way, there is a spectrum of trauma ranging from the effects of poor parenting to serious physical, emotional and mental abuse – but we also carry the unresolved traumas from our parents, grandparents, and beyond (called intergenerational trauma). We carry these traumas in our minds and bodies, often pushing them down and away – to avoid dealing with them.

We are all also plugged into our devices while facing multiple challenges in simply surviving and (ideally) thriving in our lives -- often feeling as though we have no time for ourselves, our families, our communities. Finally, adding to these woes, we are also facing a spiritual crisis, as we search for meaning and connection to a higher power.

During this same period, the pharmaceutical industry and the medical professions have collaborated to provide a wide variety of anti-anxiety pills (labeled as anxiolytics) and antidepressants. Over the last two decades, we have seen a massive increase in the long-term use of anxiolytics and antidepressant medications in the United States.

Worldwide, the global antidepressant market was valued at $15.6 billion in 2020… and is expected to reach $21 billion by 2030. In the U.S., about 1 in 5 people are on at least one antidepressant medication.

In terms of all prescription drugs, Americans filled almost **4 billion** prescriptions in 2020 – nearly 13 prescriptions for every man, woman, and child in the United States. According to the U.S. Food & Drug Administration (FDA), nearly *two-thirds of all patient visits to physicians result in one or more prescriptions.*

Sadly, many Americans have also been suffering through the opioid epidemic, moving from oxycodone to heroin to fentanyl. In the last two decades, more than a million people have died from drug overdoses – a true drug death epidemic – with the vast majority of those deaths from opioids. It should be noted that alcohol consumption and associated deaths are on the rise; in fact the U.S. Centers for Disease Control and Prevention (CDC) reports that alcohol-related deaths in the U.S. rose 30% during the years 2020 and 2021.

We are also living in a time of increased social isolation, whether from pandemics or social media or work-from-home, and many of us no longer feel a part of a community. One of the hallmarks of all psychedelics is the realization that we are all part of the human community, that we are all interconnected and interdependent. Psychedelics can actually be part of the solution to social isolation.

Suicide rates are some of the highest they have ever been – especially among veterans and first responders. Suicide is the 12th leading cause of death in the U.S., and in 2020, 45,979 people killed themselves – an average of 130 suicides per day. During that same period, about 12.2 million people seriously thought about suicide and approximately 1.2 million people attempted suicide. First responders are more likely to die by suicide than in the line of duty, and suicide is the second leading cause of death in the military community (with an estimated 22+ suicides daily). The Native American community is the worst hit by

" **INSPIRING QUOTE** "It is no surprise that psychedelics, with their activation of deeply healing intelligent capacities, seem to spontaneously engender internal and interpersonal experiences of love." – DR. ADÈLE LAFRANCE, PH.D. **"**

the suicide epidemic, having the highest suicide rate of any racial/ethnic group, with 23.9 percent of the population committing suicide, according to the U.S. Centers for Disease Control and Prevention.

More than half of Americans have reported being affected by suicide.

Finally, many people are struggling with the lack of community, connections, and spirituality typically associated with religion; many of us feel disconnected from the people and world around us. Yes, talking about religious beliefs, but spirituality is bigger than official religions: spirituality is about seeking a meaningful connection with something greater than yourself. Again, psychedelics and plant medicines have been used for centuries by people seeking a deeper connection with God, the Creator, the Divine... the Universe. And while we have been seeing a decline in organized religious affiliations, we have seen an increase in people identifying as "spiritual but not religious" (SBNR).

A recent study has shown how the pandemic (or, rather the reaction to the pandemic) has dramatically altered our personalities. The study found "significant declines in the traits that help us navigate social situations, trust others, think creatively, and act responsibly. These changes were especially pronounced among young adults."

We have been told by doctors and pharmaceutical companies (through their frequent and insidious advertising) that all we need to do to feel better is take a pill – or several pills. Often, a troubling combination of benzodiazepines (such as Xanax, Ativan, Valium, Librium, Restoril) and antidepressants (such as Wellbutrin, Lexapro, Prozac, Zoloft, Effexor, Norpramin).

What's the problem with taking a daily pill(s) for your mental health and well-being? Three problems. First, once you start taking these pills, it's often a lifetime choice and extremely difficult to wean off the medication(s). Second, many of these pills simply reduce symptoms; they are not cures but merely a temporary fix (which by default becomes a permanent "fix"). Third, many people stop taking the meds because they feel the drugs "mask" their true selves.

A recent article in *Newsweek* further explains the situation with these medications: "Evidence is mounting, however, that doctors are vastly overprescribing SSRIs. Although there is widespread agreement that SSRIs help some people with severe depression, these patients are a small minority of people who take the drugs. *"Only about 15 percent derive any more benefit from the drugs than they would a sugar pill, one recent study found."*

The good news is that emerging research is changing the way we think about depression and medicating depression. A recent study from the University College of London raises doubt on the traditional belief that a chemical imbalance in the brain is responsible for depression. Another study published in the *Journal Molecular Psychiatry* concluded that serotonin level – the target of antidepressants – is not responsible for depression.

Further good news: In the last ten years there has been a dramatic increase in the number of clinical trials testing psychedelic medicines, such as psilocybin and MDMA (with a few testing LSD and DMT), for their use in treating depression, anxiety and panic attacks, post-traumatic stress, drug dependency/addiction, and eating disorders.

Both psilocybin and MDMA have shown such positive results that many expect FDA approval for both medicines in the treatment of several conditions – initially, MDMA for post-traumatic stress and psilocybin for depression. Legal ketamine treatment clinics already exist across the U.S. and online for treatment of depression, post-traumatic stress, obsessive-compulsive disorder, and bipolar disorder – as well as to treat chronic pain and migraines.

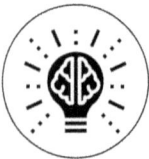

FUN FACT Psychedelic medicines are hallucinogens, used to alter and improve sensory perceptions and cognitive processes. These substances, depending on dosage, can lead to transformative and deeply spiritual experiences.

WHY THIS TOPIC?

I truly believe a major avenue for the future of healing is psychedelics, especially entheogenic plants and fungi. We have decades of research (much lost due to the "War on Drugs") on how psychedelics affect the brain… and we are seeing new studies emerging almost daily showing the positive impact of psychedelics on mood disorders (such as depression), anxiety and panic attacks, obsessive compulsive disorder (OCD), post-traumatic stress disorder (PTSD), eating disorders, addiction (to drugs, alcohol, smoking), and end-of-life anxiety.

The most recent research on psychedelics and the brain shows that these medicines help neurons in the brain grow new dendrites, which increases connections between cells – meaning psychedelics help build and solidify new circuits in the brain, allowing people to lay down more positive brain pathways. Psychedelics promote neural plasticity and increase cognition, leading to the possibility of listing psychedelics as a nootropic (a substance that supports one or more aspects of brain health and cognitive function, such as focus, mood, memory, willpower).

The problem with the current method of healing by simply using pills or the combination of pills and talk therapy is that the model is outdated and ineffective for many people. In fact, many people do not even have access to talk therapy because insurance does not cover it – but amazingly, insurance covers the pills. Others are simply wary of talking to a therapist, and wary of how many months/years they may need to be in therapy, as well as concerned about privacy issues and making a strong connection to a counselor. It should be noted, however, that talk therapy before and after a psychedelic experience (as part of preparation and integration) has shown very positive results for assisting in the healing.

Psychedelics, also referred to as hallucinogens, entheogens, or empathogens, are psychoactive substances that produce alterations in conscious experience. Traditional psychedelics (including LSD, psilocybin, mescaline, and DMT) affect the brain's serotonin system, primarily by binding to the serotonin 2A (5HT-2A) receptor. Other substances with known hallucinogenic properties (such as ketamine, MDMA, and others) have different targets in the brain but still produce some psychedelic effects.

Psychedelics, while not a miracle cure, do have the potential of helping people cut through all the layers of protective coverings to get at the root cause of the trauma, the root of the anxiety, fear, and depression. Psychedelics are a window to our souls – a window into things we have suppressed so deeply that we do not consciously understand or remember.

We have the potential for true and complete healing, and the unearthing of our authentic self, free of the hurt, anger, shame, fear. Psychedelic medicines are mind-altering substances that produce changes in perception, mood/emotions, and cognitive processes, resulting in deeper self-awareness and knowledge of who we are.

The book is also about clarifying some misconceptions about these psychedelic medicines and providing as much information and details about people's actual experiences with them – in healing, in transformation, in deepening spirituality.

INSPIRING QUOTE "Something is being born right now. In the middle of all this terrible pain and suffering, which is raging all around us, we are learning something; we're finding a deeper level of our humanity. A realization that we are all brothers and sisters who are suffering together."
– KAT (KATHLEEN) HARRISON

These are amazing and powerful stories of healing and transformation – through them and your own research, the hope is that you will one day have your own story of healing.

WHY NOW?

We are in a mental health epidemic. People are struggling more than ever before – according to the Substance Abuse and Mental Health Services Administration, with 52.9 million adults reporting any mental illness and 14.2 million adults reporting a serious mental illness in 2020. Furthermore, the National Institute of Mental Health reports that in 2020, 21 million adults in the U.S. had at least one major depressive episode.

In November 2022, Dr. Vivek Murthy, the U.S. Surgeon General, stated that the mental health crisis is the biggest concern facing the country.

We are also, not coincidentally, amidst a psychedelic renaissance – perhaps even a psychedelic revolution – and it's about time. Research in the field is booming, media interest is reaching a crescendo… and, according to a YouGovAmerica study, one in four Americans say they have tried at least one psychedelic.

Even elite athletes and entertainers are now announcing their use of – and healing with – psychedelics for medicinal, mental health and other personal reasons. Perhaps the most widely read account is of NFL Quarterback Aaron Rogers, who has stated that Ayahuasca, which he consumed in March 2020 in Peru, has helped increase his "self-love." His story appeared in *Sports Illustrated*. Other celebrities who have expressed relief and healing from psychedelics includes entertainers Joe Rogan, Will Smith (and son Jayden), Susan Sarandon, Rosie Perez, Chelsea Handler, Carrie Fisher, Megan Fox, Reggie Watts, and Seth Rogan; musicians Harry Styles, Kacey Musgraves, Miley Cyrus, Paul Simon, Ben Lee, Sting, and Paul McCartney; NHL's Daniel Carcillo; NBA's Lamar Odom; and boxer Mike Tyson.

As you'll learn in Chapter 2, all psychedelics have been listed as Schedule I controlled substances since the 1970s – the highest level of control – meaning they are considered to have no current medical use and have a high potential for abuse and/or addiction. Schedule I drugs include LSD, mescaline, MDMA, psilocybin, DMT, Ibogaine, Ayahuasca, and cannabis – but also heroin, quaaludes, bath salts. Oddly, cocaine, meth, and fentanyl are all Schedule II drugs.

Ketamine (perhaps because of its primary use as an anesthetic) is listed as a Schedule III drug. Interesting to note that two of the most abused drugs in their use – alcohol and tobacco/nicotine – are not even included in this list.

Let that last statement sit for a minute… the two deadliest and most abused drugs are not even considered drugs that need to be on the controlled substance list.

Psychedelics are still illegal in the U.S. at the Federal level, but we are quickly moving from a black-and- white approach to one with lots of grey areas – loosening the consequences for personal use or small, noncommercial amounts of psychedelics. Still, this book is not about encouraging illegal drug use. It's about showcasing the many benefits of these medicines. Please move forward accordingly – and with caution. The focus of this book is education and empowerment.

All across the country, numerous municipalities and state legislatures are considering and/or passing laws that at a minimum decriminalize psychedelics, while others are looking at complete legalization – and still others are allowing medical/research use. (Many of these strategies follow the cannabis playbook.) Oregon has led the way at the state level, followed by Colorado – with the cities of Denver, Oakland, Santa Cruz, and Ann Arbor making dramatic changes within city limits.

66 **INSPIRING QUOTE** "Psilocybin not only produces significant and immediate effects, it also has a long duration, which suggests that it may be a uniquely useful new treatment for depression." – ROLAND GRIFFITHS, PH.D. **99**

There are also numerous grassroots groups organizing efforts to remove the stigma of these amazing psychedelics, many of which are plants. Perhaps the best-known group is *Decriminalize Nature*, whose mission is about "decriminalizing and expanding access to entheogenic plants and fungi through political and community organizing, education and advocacy." (Entheogenic includes Ibogaine, dimethyltryptamine/DMT, mescaline, psilocybin/psilocyn, LSD.)

One of the oldest and most respected organizations leading the research on psychedelics, especially with MDMA, is MAPS – the Multidisciplinary Association for Psychedelic Studies – whose mission as a nonprofit research and educational organization is to develop medical, legal, and cultural contexts for people to benefit from the careful uses of psychedelics and cannabis. And while the MDMA research has received the most media attention and excitement (with FDA approval expected in the next year or so), MAPS also conducted clinical research on Ayahuasca (with a focus on it treating drug addiction), LSD (for treatment of anxiety with people with life-threatening illnesses), Ibogaine (for treatment of opioid and alcohol addiction), and cannabis (for treatment of PTSD in war veterans). The organization's vision: "We envision a world where psychedelics and marijuana are safely and legally available for beneficial uses, and where research is governed by rigorous scientific evaluation of their risks and benefits."

Another organization leading the research charge with psychedelics is the Beckley Foundation, which has conducted studies with cannabis, psilocybin (for treatment-resistant depression), LSD (for treatment of anxiety and mood disorders), MDMA, and Ayahuasca (for treatment of depression, anxiety, grief and PTSD). Its mission is twofold: first, to investigate the effects of psychoactive substances on the brain and consciousness in order to harness their potential benefits and minimize their potential harms; second, to achieve evidence-based changes in global drug policies so to reduce the harms brought about by the unintended negative consequences of current drug policies; and develop improved policies based on health, harm reduction, cost-effectiveness, and human rights.

Several universities are also leading the way in the clinical research, including Johns Hopkins, Washington University, Harvard University, Stanford University, Yale University, University of Utah, New York University, UC Berkeley, Northwestern University, University of Pittsburgh, UT Houston, UT Austin, University of Wisconsin-Madison, University of Saskatchewan, the Imperial College of London, and many others (https://psychedelicinvest.com/educational-organizations/).

Even some companies are getting behind the healing effects of these psychedelic medicines. The best example is a brand you may not be that familiar with (as it is more often found in natural health stores) called Dr. Bronner's, a company founded in the 1940s in the U.S. and known as a producer of organic and environmentally-responsible soap and personal care products that dedicates its profits to making a better world. Today, some of those profits – more than $3 million so far – are being used to urge the FDA to consider the legalization of medical psychedelics to aid in the treatment of mental health through the company's *Heal Soul* campaign. (The label on the company's 32-ounce soap aims to educate the public about these life-saving therapies and medicines, and the advocacy organizations and ballot initiatives that are advancing this work.)

Finally, it is simply time to reconfigure and change our thoughts on "drug" safety and recognize that there are many more dangerous and lethal drugs than psychedelics, which have a very low death rate. In fact, more than 700,000 people die annually from "legal" drugs… Deaths per year:

- 500,000 deaths related to tobacco
- 100,000 deaths related to alcohol
- 92,000 deaths from illicit drug overdoses
- 30,000+ deaths related to pharmaceuticals
- <20 deaths related to psychedelics

One more sobering statistic: prescription drugs are the *third leading cause of death* after heart disease and cancer in the United States and Europe, with another 2 million people also suffering from non-fatal adverse reactions tied to prescription drugs that have been deemed safe by the FDA. According to the research, about half of those who die have taken their prescriptions correctly; the other half die because of errors, such as too high a dose or use of a drug despite contraindications.

WHY ME?

I have been an educator and writer for all my life, for many years focused mostly on my discipline of marketing – but over the last two decades slowly moving to fields in which I have more passion. These fields include health and wellness, focused mainly on what we eat, how we exercise, and getting out into nature.

My focus is on empowering people to live better, healthier lives.

Several years ago, my wife Jenny happened to be listening to a podcast featuring Jesse Gould, a former Army Ranger who spent years following his return to the states from tours in the Middle East struggling – not sleeping well, the lack of support from the Veterans Administration (which simply pushed pills to deal with these issues), self-medicating to tamp down his demons. Through his desperation, he found out about Ayahuasca and the stories of tremendous healing. He took a shot and found his own healing through the medicine and integration. This experience led him to found the nonprofit, Heroic Hearts Project (HHP), whose mission is to build a healing community that helps veterans suffering from military trauma recover and thrive by providing them with safe, supervised access to psychedelic treatments, professional coaching, and ongoing peer support.

" **INSPIRING QUOTE** "In the kind of world we have today, transformation of humanity might well be our only real hope for survival." – STANISLAV GROF, MD, PH.D. **"**

11

Jenny was so moved by Jesse's story and the mission of HHP that she immediately contacted him and asked how she could help. Once she got involved with HHP, that led to her deepening involvement in the psychedelic movement – and we both became immersed into the field of plant medicines and psychedelics. Jenny now also works for Psychedelic Passage, a leader in helping people connect with trained psychedelic facilitators across the country for safe and healing journeys.

I bring together my research skills, my educational abilities, and my desire to help and empower to this book. But even beyond these elements, I have also participated in psychedelic healing and spiritual journeys with MDMA, psilocybin, LSD, and Ayahuasca – in various settings. I am connected with hundreds of people who are working and healing in the psychedelic space.

> **INSPIRING QUOTE** "Psychedelics open a door and provide an opportunity... For the best results you need a desire for personal and spiritual growth, even if it entails some degree of suffering." – WILLIAM (BILL) RICHARDS, PH.D.

WHY YOU?

Why are you here? My hope is you are seeking healing for yourself and/or a loved one. Trauma is the invisible force that profoundly affects many of our lives. How we act today is often deeply influenced by our reactions to the wounds we have suffered in the past.

What is trauma? Addiction specialist and best-selling author Dr. Gabor Maté discusses the two kinds of trauma in his latest book, *The Myth of Normal*: horrible things done to us is the most common we think about, but trauma can also be the withholding of attention, kindness, love.

We have **all** experienced trauma in our lives. Dr. Paul Conti, psychologist, trauma expert, and author of *Trauma: The Invisible Epidemic*, states that trauma is an unseen epidemic, affecting us all … "it can hijack your entire body without notice. It can transfer easily between parent and child. If left untreated, it can perniciously erode and denigrate every aspect of your life. It can last a lifetime. And – unless confronted and healed – can come with a potentially fatal prognosis."

Then, there's also trauma that gets passed down from one generation to another, called intergenerational trauma. Professor of Psychiatry and Neuroscience Dr. Rachel Yehuda is a leading researcher, studying PTSD and intergenerational trauma (also called Transgenerational trauma) for years, specifically researching holocaust survivors and their children.

Finally, your lifelong efforts to block or ignore these traumatic events is most likely exacting a toll on you, whether you are aware or not. According to best-selling author (of *Your Body Keeps Score*), psychiatrist, and neuroscientist Dr. Bessel van der Kolk, "the problem with trauma is that when it is over, your body continues to relive it." Trauma, he notes, is not the thing that happens to us, but how we respond to that event – and it changes your brain, permanently. Note that stress and potential negative aspects of everyday life add to that stored trauma.

While this trauma may not kill us, according to Dr. Peter A. Levine (in his book, *Healing Trauma: A Pioneering Program for Restoring the Wisdom of Your Body*), "if we do not resolve it, our lives can be severely diminished by its effects. Some people have even described this situation as a "living death."

Of course, you may also be interested in psychedelics to simply help expand your mind and break out of a creative or emotional funk. Perhaps you are simply seeking a mystical or spiritual experience.

If you are seeking knowledge and firsthand accounts of other people's authentic psychedelic experiences and healing, then this is the book for you. This book is not meant for recreational users, but people seeking transformation through intentional (and some would say sacred) use of psychedelic substances.

The book contains stories – personal narratives – from as many different types of people as possible, especially those in the BIPOC community, who continue to be greatly underrepresented in using these psychedelic medicines, with women and Black women severely unrepresented.

These stories are not meant to be beautifully flowing narratives or trip reports. Instead, the goal is to show you all the details of the different types of psychedelic experiences – whether using magic mushrooms (psilocybin) or mescaline or LSD or DMT – from the words of people who have taken these journeys and can share the impact of the medicines on themselves.

Psychedelics are NOT for everyone, but they are, in general, very safe medicines – certainly safer than alcohol and tobacco. If you are open to them, these compounds can offer you physical, psychological, and spiritual healing. Many of these medicines are also heart-opening, making you more receptive to what you see and learn from the journey.

"

INSPIRING QUOTE "When I told Michael Pollan that psilocybin mushrooms changed my mind, I meant that literally; I think they built new neural pathways in my brain that allowed me to articulate my thoughts more clearly and to become a more creative and more peaceful person." – PAUL STAMETS **"**

People need to be fairly physically healthy and mentally sound when taking psychedelics – no serious heart or respiratory conditions. The biggest concern is people with schizophrenia or with schizophrenic tendencies, who may experience a psychotic break from a psychedelic experience. There is a concern of negative impact for bipolar and personality disorders, although these populations have not been adequately studied.

Otherwise, psychedelics are safe – hard/impossible to overdose and not additive – but if you are taking certain medications, you will need to consult with experts on the best way to proceed; these experts and organizations are listed in the back of the book. Finally, psychedelics are not recommended for women who are pregnant or breastfeeding.

Most importantly, you MUST be willing to do the work. The medicine will interact with you and show you what is wrong; the trauma you experienced but had forgotten, what needs to be fixed, even how to fix these things, but the medicine – the psychedelic experience – **is just the beginning of a long journey of healing and work** on changing your life. We call this "after" process **integration**, and it will be covered in detail later in the book.

Generally speaking, these psychedelic medicines work best if you are:

- *Open to the concept of psychedelics as medicine;*
- *Prepared to face whatever the medicine has to show you;*
- *Clear that these medicines are not magic pills, but part of a process of healing;*
- *Ready to make fundamental changes to your life;*
- *Committed to letting go, being open-minded, and surrendering to the medicine;*
- *Willing to step into the unknown and down the rabbit hole;*
- *Excited about the possibility of true healing (along with potential spiritual growth);*
- *Dedicated to the proper preparation and integration required.*

Most people who have taken one of these psychedelic medicines report back that the experience was one of the most powerful and novel experiences of their lives – categorizing the psychedelic journey as one of the top five pivotal moments of their lives – on the same magnitude as the birth of a child, the death of a parent.

WHAT THIS BOOK IS – AND IS NOT

This book is about healing, about spiritual and personal growth. It's about educating and empowering you. It is not about the recreational use of psychedelics, but instead taking these medicines for life transformation… and, believe me, when these medicines are used with *respect and intention*, the transformations are absolutely amazing, beautiful, life-saving.

The core of this book is sharing the details of people's experiences with psychedelics so that you can have a stronger sense of what to expect – and what not to expect – on your psychedelic journey. But do take these stories with a grain of salt, as everyone's experiences with the medicines are unique.

Everyone knows that psychedelics are "trippy." Yes, you might see interesting visuals and geometric patterns during part of your psychedelic experience, but that's not why people take these medicines, and it is also not guaranteed that you will have any visuals.

This book is about educating you on the different types of psychedelic medicines and experiences – through the lens of others just like you. It is a book for people new to these medicines and seeking further knowledge.

The book is not meant to be a detailed history of these drugs, nor a scientific study of exactly how these medicines work in our brain; there are other books about psychedelics that cover their history and their effects on the brain, and you can find a list of those resources at the end of the book.

This book focuses on true psychedelics and hallucinogens, and has purposely omitted cannabis, which most do <u>not</u> consider a psychedelic (though some strains/combinations do have psychoactive properties). It is also not included as most studies find it is used more recreationally than for treatment of mental health conditions or spiritual growth.

Finally, if the thought of hallucinogenic psychedelics is a bit too overwhelming for you, a trend in recent years is microdosing these psychedelic medicines – microdosing in such small amounts that you gain the benefits from the medicine without the hallucinating effects from the macrodoses. You'll find more about microdosing in Chapter 24.

INSPIRING QUOTE "I think of going to the grave without having a psychedelic experience like going to the grave without ever having sex. It means that you never figured out what it is all about. The mystery is in the body and the way the body works itself into nature." -TERENCE MCKENNA

DISCLAIMER

As of this writing, all psychedelics – in the United States – are illegal. Yes, there are some small pockets of cities (and two states) that have decriminalized small amounts of psychedelics for personal use. And yes, there are clinical trials that may lead to MDMA and psilocybin being FDA-approved for therapeutic uses. BUT, if you do not plan to leave the U.S. for your psychedelic experience, you face some difficult (and perhaps impossible) choices in how you find and source the medicine for your healing.

Until psychedelics become mainstream in some fashion, you will face the possibility of legal consequences if you seek healing.

You should also be aware that if you decide to do one of these medicines in the U.S., you have several options – from using a healing center to working with a psychedelic-assisted therapist to working with a trained facilitator/tripsitter. Whichever avenue you pursue, please do it with caution – or seek only legal treatments, such as ketamine in the U.S. (or a clinical trial with MDMA, psilocybin, or LSD), or a healing center in some of the few places where some of these medications are legal (such as Ayahuasca in Costa Rica, Mexico, and Peru).

EXTRAS

As you work your way through the book, you'll encounter some extra bits of information that I believe you will find helpful as you make your journey through the beautiful and amazing stories of healing through these psychedelic medicines.

Here's what to expect:

- *Fun Facts:* Key bits of trivia and information
- *Inspiring Quotes:* Helpful quotes from key psychedelic heroes and leaders
- *Pitfalls to Healing:* Occasional warnings about issues to avoid
- *Facilitator Tips:* Useful suggestions for managing a safe trip

PROCEEDS FROM THIS BOOK

All proceeds from the sale of this book (minus costs) will be donated to several very worthy nonprofit organizations in the psychedelic space, including Chacruna Institute and Heroic Hearts Project.

PART ONE:
THE BASICS
OF PSYCHEDELIC
MEDICINES

WELCOME

This section of the book is designed to provide you with a broad overview of psychedelics and psychedelic medicines, from their early uses to the present day.

The goal here is to provide enough information about the history and uses of these medicines so you can make an informed choice – or start on a path to discovering more information.

In a later section, a list of books and documentaries is provided so that you can delve deeper into the subject, including books on each of the major psychedelics.

After this section comes 20 chapters of healing and transformative stories – from a wide variety of people.

CHAPTER ONE
Frequently Asked Questions About Psychedelics

Here is a collection of the most commonly asked questions about psychedelics. Find your answers here, as well as in more detail in the rest of the book.

1. SHOULDN'T I "JUST SAY NO" TO PSYCHEDELICS?

Any medical/health choice is yours to make, but eliminating perhaps one of the best classes of medicines (many of which are natural substances) simply because of 50 years of propaganda would be a shame.

These medicines are finally getting the detailed research they deserve, and most of the results are astounding – and unexpected. Consuming psychedelic medicine with intent is seeing tremendous results in clinical trials, further supported by thousands of years of use by Indigenous people around the globe.

As discussed in Chapter 3, psychedelics are being hailed as a key tool in the battle against depression and mood disorders, anxiety, control disorders (eating, OCD), addiction (alcohol, opioids), and more.

2. AREN'T PSYCHEDELICS JUST RECREATIONAL?

While there will always be people who take drugs for their recreational value, after decades of misinformation, scientists and clinic studies around the world are

INSPIRING QUOTE "Psychedelics are illegal not because a loving government is concerned that you may jump out of a third story window. Psychedelics are illegal because they dissolve opinion structures and culturally laid down models of behavior and information processing. They open you up to the possibility that everything you know is wrong."
–TERENCE MCKENNA

publishing promising results for the potential these medicines have in a variety of areas, including:

- *Post-traumatic stress (PTS)*
- *Depression and mood disorders*
- *Anxiety*
- *Addictions (smoking, drinking, opioids)*
- *Control disorders (eating, OCD)*
- *Cluster headaches, migraines*
- *Furthermore, these medicines are also being used for spiritual awakenings and transformational learning.*

INSPIRING QUOTE "This is the most powerful drug I have ever experienced. Yage is not like anything else. It produces the most complete derangement of the senses."
– WILLIAM BURROUGHS

3. HOW CAN PSYCHEDELICS HELP ME?

These psychedelic medicines can be truly transformative. They are tools that you can use to face hidden (and not so hidden) traumas, demons, and negative thoughts/feelings – and remove the negative effects those things are causing in your life.

These psychedelic medicines will show you exactly what needs to be healed within you – and then it's up to you, through a process we call integration, to heal yourself and move forward with your life.

Psychedelics are not just for mental healing, but spiritual healing and awakening as well. At higher doses of these medicines, people report talking with angels, Jesus, and even God/The Creator itself.

Finally, if you are seeking clarity or trying to find novel and unique solutions to a complex problem, then these psychedelic medicines can also help you uncover unique solutions.

4. ARE PSYCHEDELICS SAFE?

What is safe? If you are taking any prescription drugs, are they safe? As you'll see in Chapter 2, psychedelic medicines are not recommended for everyone, but they are much safer than most prescription drugs (with their ridiculous lists of side effects). Psychedelics are much safer than alcohol and tobacco, let alone the various street drugs.

People with certain mental conditions (such as those with schizophrenic tendencies) and those with physical health conditions (such as breathing, heart issues) should not consume psychedelic medicines. People taking certain prescriptions for depression/mood disorders/anxiety may need to taper down the dosages to get the best effects from the psychedelics (with adequate medical/mental health supervision).

5. ARE ALL PSYCHEDELICS THE SAME?

Yes and no. For simplicity, experts have decided to list eight major psychedelics. (In reality, there may be an almost infinite number of psychoactive and hallucinogenic drugs that can be synthesized in the lab.)

Of those eight psychedelic medicines, six are considered classic psychedelics – also serotonergic psychedelics, meaning these substances work by activating the 5HT2A receptors, causing shifts in perception, potential ego death/dissolution, and introspection. These medicines include LSD, psilocybin, DMT, Ayahuasca, Ibogaine, and mescaline.

The other two main "psychedelics" – ketamine and MDMA – are in their own classes. Ketamine is a NMDA-based dissociative, which works by blocking NMDA receptors. MDMA is classified as an empathogen, a class of substances that are able to elicit strong feelings of empathy in users.

Learn more about each substance in Chapters 2 and 3.

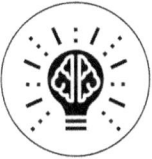

FUN FACT Feelings of unconditional, non-judgmental love are among the most common experiences people report after taking these psychedelic medicines – and love is an essential healing modality. We all need love.

6. CAN SOMEONE OVERDOSE ON PSYCHEDELICS?

The short answer is that you can overdose on anything – if you try hard enough.

Believe it or not, the true psychedelics (LSD, psilocybin, mescaline, DMT, Ibogaine, Ayahuasca) are some of the safest drugs available; in fact, if you have nutmeg at home for baking, it has the potential to be much more harmful if overconsumed compared to a psychedelic.

Ketamine and MDMA, while safe in controlled doses, are slightly different than traditional psychedelics.

7. AM I SIMPLY TRADING ONE DRUG ADDICTION FOR ANOTHER?

No. People usually ask this question in regard to the power of psychedelic medicines to have a dramatic impact on breaking addiction.

Unlike alcohol and street drugs (such as heroin, cocaine, meth, etc.), these psychedelic medicines are not addictive and the vast majority of people taking them with intention do so for healing – and at the doses many take, there is no interest or need to continue consuming.

Of course, almost anything can be the focus of an addiction, and if any psychedelics have a higher chance of repeated use – recreationally – it would be MDMA and ketamine.

8. HOW CAN I GO ABOUT TAKING A PSYCHEDELIC MEDICINE?

It depends – and it will probably depend for many years into the future as the psychedelic landscape continues to evolve, ideally with several of these medicines being reclassified as medicinal and therapeutic.

That said, you have four options for completing an intentional psychedelic experience.

- *Complete treatment at a clinical trial*
- *Complete treatment at a legal healing center/retreat center*
- *Complete treatment using an underground healing center (not advised)*
- *Complete treatment on your own, purchasing from an underground seller (not advised)*

Things to know. Trials are well underway for MDMA and psilocybin. LSD has just started back in clinical trials. Ketamine is legally available at clinics (including several that offer telehealth services) around the country. Ayahuasca, Ibogaine, and psilocybin are legal in a very small number of countries. Mescaline is an official sacrament of the Native American Church (and thus legal for members).

FACILITATOR TIP If you are considering a solo macrodose psychedelic journey, experts strongly suggest starting with a low dose for your first experience, gradually increasing the dosage in future journeys – as needed for healing.

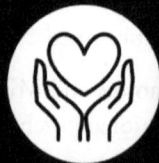

9. HOW CAN I SOURCE PSYCHEDELIC MEDICINES?

Perhaps the toughest question to answer – for a variety of reasons.

Most of these psychedelic medicines are currently classified as illegal at the U.S. federal level (making them illegal everywhere except small pockets of places that have moved to decriminalize small amounts of the substances). Thus, go into this whole process with open eyes.

First, you could legally consume these psychedelic medicines by participating in one of several scientific trials occurring around the country.

Second, some suppliers are operating in the gray market, but many more are completely underground, making private sourcing a tough issue. And, of course, there are scammers pretending to sell these medicines. Consider joining a psychedelic society, where members may be able to recommend reputable sources.

Third, there are places around the world where these substances are legal, thus you could travel to these places to source and hold ceremony.

Fourth, there are underground healing centers, facilities, and "churches" offering psychedelic medicine ceremonies.

> **INSPIRING QUOTE** "I believe it's true to say that everyone who has experienced LSD or another psychedelic would look on that experience, especially the first one, as a major life-changing event." – RALPH METZNER, PH.D.

10. WHAT IS THE BEST PSYCHEDELIC MEDICINE FOR NEWBIES?

Certainly the most popular and widely used psychedelic medicine is psilocybin, since there are hundreds of varieties of "magic" mushrooms growing around the world. The duration of the experience is also not too long – sort of in the middle for all psychedelics (approximately 4-5 hours).

Of the class psychedelics, mescaline might be the next best for first-timers, as the medicine is fairly mild and very heart-opening.

Finally, MDMA is also extremely heart-opening – with few of the hallucinations/visions associated with the other psychedelics.

Read more about the effects of these psychedelics in Chapters 2 and 3.

11. WHAT ARE THE DANGERS OF CONSUMING PSYCHEDELICS?

These medicines are extremely safe – when the substances are properly consumed, meaning the medicine has been properly and safely sourced and the dosage carefully measured, and set and setting established.

If you are mentally and physically well/stable, these medicines have little or no side effects – especially when compared to pharmaceutical drugs, which often have a litany of dangerous conditions and side effects.

The plant-based psychedelics (psilocybin, Ayahuasca, Ibogaine) have been safely consumed by Indigenous people for thousands of years. LSD is derived from ergot (a fungus that grows naturally on grains); ergot also has been used for centuries to produce psychedelic beers and wines.

Of course, before making any changes, people should consult with their doctors – especially those with health issues.

12. WHAT CAN I EXPECT WHEN TAKING A PSYCHEDELIC MEDICINE?

Each medicine has different aspects, including intensity and duration length, so your first step should be understanding what to expect with the medicine you have chosen to use – and the dosage you will be consuming.

With all these medications, there is a ramp up after ingestion that includes mostly physical characteristics – including temperature fluctuations, sensitivity to light and sound, and often nausea. During the peak period of the medicine, expect to have visual patterns and distortions with possible hallucinations (with eyes open or closed, depending on dosage); deep insights and images of the past; conversations with yourself or other beings; and be transported by the music; you may also encounter an out-of-body experience. During the come down, you may slowly get your appetite back; more insights will continue to flow; and you may experience a feeling of joy or satisfaction… even Zen.

After the journey, it is important to hydrate and eat, as well as rest your brain.

> **INSPIRING QUOTE** "For me, 'spiritual' is a good name for some of the powerful mental phenomena that arise when the voice of the ego is muted or silenced. If nothing else, these journeys have shown me how that psychic construct—at once so familiar and on reflection so strange—stands between us and some striking new dimensions of experience, whether of the world outside us or of the mind within." – MICHAEL POLLAN

13. SHOULD I BE AFRAID OF HAVING A BAD TRIP?

Get that bad trip image out of your head – those so-called "bad trips" we witnessed in anti-drug advertising and movies is total propaganda. As long as you are healthy and follow proper procedures for an intentional healing journey using a psychedelic medicine, you will not die nor will you lose your mind.

A better question might be, should I be afraid of what I might encounter during a journey? The answer is still a no, but you should be prepared to face some challenging issues/images/memories.

We talk about challenging trips, not bad trips. And yes, you may be faced with some challenging issues, some intense visions – but you need to face these things for healing to occur. It's also because of the possible challenges, that most people recommend that you take these medicines in situations where you will have support – support from a clinician, facilitator, tripsitter, or sober friend.

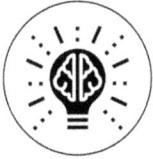

FUN FACT Love is a wonderful and recurrent theme in psychedelic journeys; yes, it's about facing our challenges, our traumas, but always in a loving, nurturing way. Love is truly all around us – especially during a psychedelic journey.

14. HOW CAN I ENSURE THAT I HAVE A GOOD TRIP?

Preparation and intention. With psychedelic medicines, best practices include what's called set and setting, which is covered in detail in Chapter 3.

It should be noted that there are no guarantees for a "good" or successful trip; that said, the more preparation you do beforehand, the more likely you will have the kind of journey you are hoping for.

Set: Shorthand for mindset – and it's all about being mentally prepared for your psychedelic medicine journey. This term is about setting a goal or intention for your journey; what you hope to accomplish/discover/experience. It also covers the all-important mindset of surrendering to the medicine. One of the top reasons for not achieving a successful journey is when participants do not fully surrender to the medicine – and the deeper a thinker you are, the harder it will be to fully surrender.

Setting: This term deals with your feelings of comfort and safety in the location in which you will consume the medicine. If you go to a clinic or healing center, the setting should be firmly established. If you are planning to do a personal journey, then it's about finding the best and most comfortable and conducive spot – for you.

Finally, preparation also involves eating and living as cleanly as possible for at least a week before your psychedelic experience.

15. CAN I TAKE A PSYCHEDELIC WHEN I AM ALONE? WHAT IS A TRIP SITTER? DO I NEED ONE?

Yes, you can, but it is ill-advised to do so when ingesting large doses of the medicine.

This question is not as simple as it looks – and neither is the answer. For very low doses and microdosing, there is no real need for a tripsitter, though some people still hire one.

For your first macrodosing journey, most recommend having at a minimum, a sober friend who knows what you are doing and will watch over you. If no one is available, or you would rather have an experienced professional, then you should consider hiring a tripsitter – a facilitator/guide who will sit with you as you journey through the medicine.

At higher doses, unless you are extremely experienced, you should always have someone with you.

> **" INSPIRING QUOTE** "Part of the way you change people's minds is by sharing stories of healing… Everyone has a role to play in the shaping of this movement." – AMY EMERSON, PH.D. **"**

16. I HAVE HEARD OF BRAINS BEING FRIED AND BIRTH DEFECTS FROM PSYCHEDELICS. TRUE?

No truth whatsoever; both claims were part of the disinformation campaign from the *War on Drugs*.

The more recent studies of the effects of psychedelics on the brain are positive and exciting… and they show that psychedelics can improve and help the brain heal. Psychedelics are seen to increase neuroplasticity, meaning that these medicines help release damaging habits and negative associations by building new connections within and across the brain.

In some rare cases (mostly studied with LSD, although also with psilocybin), some people experience Hallucinogen Persisting Perception Disorder (HPPD), a non-psychotic disorder that involves seeing hallucinations, halos, flashbacks, and which usually resolves within a year. The key is knowing that the possibility exists, and understanding that it is typically temporary.

Birth defects? No. Scare tactics. Recent studies from scientists around the world prove that psychedelics do not cause any genetic damage and birth defects.

17. WHAT ARE INTENTIONS – AND WHY DO I NEED THEM?

As we discuss in some detail in Chapter 3, setting intentions is one of the essential preparation steps in preparing for a successful psychedelic experience.

Intentions are about clearly stating your motivation for your psychedelic journey – and help keep us focused on the concept that we should be taking an active part in setting the direction of our experience.

Intentions can be fairly open and general, such as "show me what part of me needs healing."

Intentions can also be very specific, such as "Help me heal from my childhood sexual abuse" or "Help me break my addiction to alcohol."

What should your intention be? Start with the big question – the why. Why are you embarking on a psychedelic medicine journey? What are you hoping to accomplish? What negative elements/thinking do you want to eliminate? What kind of transformation are you seeking? Are you seeking a deeper connection to the world – to a divine being?

But do know that even with a solid intention, the medicine is going to show you what it knows you need to see. Be prepared to roll with whatever happens during your journey.

18. WHAT IS INTEGRATION – AND WHY DO I NEED IT?

Without integration, you are simply wasting time and money taking psychedelics – or basically doing so for more recreational purposes.

Integration, as discussed in Chapter 3, is about making sense of your psychedelic experience.

Integration is an integral part of figuring out how to incorporate the lessons learned from your psychedelic journey into your life, figuring out how to heal

PITFALLS TO HEALING While many of these psychedelic medicines affect the brain in similar ways, not every one will work on your brain, so it is very important to find the medicine that resonates and works best for you and your health/wellness goals.

from any previously unknown traumas, figuring out what all the images you saw mean, what the whole experience means.

Most people integrate through journaling – either electronically or with pen and paper. Others paint, draw, create. The process you use is not nearly as important as doing the work.

You can do most of your integrating by yourself, contemplating all that you discovered in your journey, or, you can integrate with others – including hiring an integration coach and/or finding a community of like-minded people.

Integration is an on-going process – and some would say a lifelong process.

INSPIRING QUOTE "Why would having an Ayahuasca experience appeal to anyone? I think people are searching for some degree of a psycho spiritual transformation." – CHARLES GROB, MD.

19. WHAT IF I DON'T WANT TO HALLUCINATE, BUT DO WANT HEALING?

Numerous companies within the psychedelics industry are developing and/or testing versions of these medicines that can still have the healing benefits without the hallucinations.

A non-hallucinogenic psychedelic medicine could be the breakthrough that truly transforms the healthcare system and brings psychedelic medicines into the mainstream.

Do your research… these medicines are coming online soon. And without the hallucinations, psychedelics could become even more widespread, eliminating the need for clinics, tripsitters, and more.

That said, do not shy away from the complete psychedelic experience… the power of these psychedelics to open the mind and heart are truly unique and amazing – profound experiences that are always touted as one of the "top five" experiences of people's lives.

One other option is to consider microdosing with a psychedelic medicine.

20. WHAT IS MICRODOSING?

Microdosing, discussed in detail in Chapter 24, is consuming an extremely low dose of a psychedelic medicine. Microdosing is another option of using these medicines – without having to worry about the hallucinogenic aspects of a full-on, full-dose journey.

To be clear, with microdosing, you can get the benefits of the medicine without getting the "psychedelic" experience.

The idea behind microdosing is to encourage an increased state of perception and calm, rather than going into a hallucinating state. Thus, microdosing is taking a minuscule dose of the medicine… so small that you will not have any hallucinations or even feel "high."

People are microdosing psychedelics to help deal with anxiety and depression – while others are doing so for an increase in productivity, to enhance perception, to sharpen focus, to deepen levels of creativity, to foster spiritual growth. Most of the success stories with microdosing are self-reported and anecdotal, but more quantitative research is being conducted.

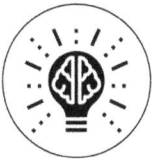 **FUN FACT** Many people believe that we are called to the medicine – especially so with the psychedelic plants and fungi. That rather than chasing down a psychedelic experience, one should wait until being summoned by the medicine.

BONUS: ISN'T CANNABIS A PSYCHEDELIC?

While cannabis is most definitely a master plant that is worthy of study and medicinal use, – one that can even have some psychoactive properties – most experts do not consider cannabis to be a psychedelic. That said, research is discovering amazing benefits from cannabis, especially in relation to post-traumatic stress, inflammation, anxiety, pain, and sleep issues.

Finally, the differences between psychedelics and cannabis are clear. People report taking psychedelics for the purpose of healing and transformation, while many people report taking cannabis recreationally (and less for healing). For the vast majority of people, psychedelics are taken with intention, not recreationally.

FACILITATOR TIP The two best sources for finding locations where people can legally ingest these medicines are Retreat.guru for healing centers and ClinicalTrials.gov for research studies needing participants.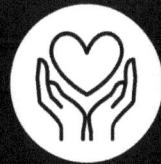

FACILITATOR TIP Consuming any psychedelic medicine can lead to unpleasant feelings and visions – the components of a challenging experience (the so-called "bad trip"). But even deep into a journey, people have the ability to "swipe left" and make the journey move away from those bad feelings and back to healing.

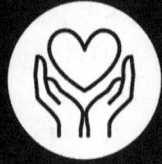

BONUS: IS THERE A CHECKLIST FOR CONSUMING PSYCHEDELICS AT HOME?

Sure. Here's a sample checklist of materials and things you should have at hand before you start an intentional psychedelic medicine journey:

- *Medicine (verified purity, dosage)*
- *Relaxing, private, and safe sitting/lounging space*
- *Comfortable, loose clothing (or naked if you like)*
- *Cozy blankets, pillows*
- *Integration supplies (journal, paper, pens, paints, recorder, etc.)*
- *Water, juice, electrolytes*
- *Snacks*
- *Tissues*
- *Headphones (optional)*
- *Eye covering/mask (optional)*
- *Music selection (timed to length of journey)*
- *Bucket (for purging)*
- *Phone (silenced, but nearby for emergencies)*
- *Sober friend or tripsitter/facilitator/ceremonialist*
- *Intentions/mantra*

CHAPTER TWO

The Real Psychedelic Revolution and Its Historical Context

In the United States, we are in the second and most widespread psychedelic movement ever known. Maybe it's a coincidence, but perhaps it's the reason, we are also in the midst of the largest mental health crisis ever experienced. Numerous factors have led us to this point – social isolation, social media, health crises (including the pandemic) – to a tipping point.

Unlike the first psychedelic revolution of the 1960s and 1970s, which was driven primarily by recreational use (especially with magic mushrooms and LSD), this current renaissance is being driven by scientific research into how these medicines affect the brain and how they may be amazing tools for healing a variety of ailments, including depression, anxiety and panic attacks, control disorders (such as OCD and eating disorders), post-traumatic stress disorder (PTSD), and addiction.

Cities, states, and even the Federal Government are contemplating revising how we view our "drug policy" – deciding whether these psychedelics, all plant medicines, or even all drugs should be decriminalized or legalized – or whether we keep the status quo. It's an ever-changing, but interesting landscape.

That said, all psychedelics are still illegal at the federal level and in most states. Thus, if you choose to take healing into your own hands, you will be breaking the law – first by purchasing the medicines and then by consuming them. On the other hand, more and more clinical trials are being approved for psychedelic medicines, so that may be an option for you. Or, you can travel outside the U.S. to retreat centers in countries where psychedelics are legal.

" INSPIRING QUOTE "Psychedelic experiences are notoriously hard to render in words; to try is necessarily to do violence to what has been seen and felt, which is in some fundamental way pre- or post-linguistic or, as students of mysticism say, ineffable." – MICHAEL POLLAN **"**

PSYCHEDELIC MEDICINE HISTORY

But before we get too caught up in the present, let's take a short, but important, trip through the history of psychedelics and entheogenic plants. (If you're looking for a more detailed history of psychedelic use over time, check out this website: https://blog.retreat.guru/the-history-of-psychedelics).

PSILOCYBIN/MAGIC MUSHROOMS: More formally known as psilocybin to get away from the recreational use stigma of "magic mushrooms," fungi with psychoactive properties have been used for as many as 10,000 years – maybe even longer. Hallucinogenic mushrooms include more than 200 species that contain psychedelic substances, mainly psilocybin which turns into psilocin upon ingestion); these mushrooms can be found across the globe: 53 are found in Mexico, 22 in the United States and Canada, 19 in Australia and the surrounding islands, 16 in Europe, 15 in Asia, and 4 in Africa. (Varieties include Copelandia, Gymnopilus, Inocybe, Panaeolus, Pholiotina, Pluteus, and Psilocybe.)

Based on archeological diggings and other research, these mushrooms have been found on rock paintings from circa 9000 BC in North Africa, as well as in Mayan and Aztec ruins in southern Mexico and northern Central America and central Mexico, respectively.

For most of history, these mushrooms were consumed mostly in religious ceremonies managed by shamans (priests). Of course, there may always have been people consuming the mushrooms for recreational uses. When the Spaniards came and conquered Mexico in the 1500s, Catholic friars weren't too keen on shamanic rituals – and for more than 300 years, the Spaniards banned the use of magic mushrooms in tribal ceremonies.

The great awakening for magic mushrooms started in the 1950s when an American businessman and his wife traveled to Mexico to study mushrooms. (They had previously found hallucinogenic mushrooms on trips to the Catskills and Russia.) During the exploration, R. Gordon Wasson and his wife Valentina Pavlovna uncovered the use of mushrooms for healing and sought out María Sabina, widely regarded as the most famous and revered Mexican healer. The husband-wife duo convinced Sabina to take them on a healing journey. The experiences were so powerful that both wrote about them in 1957 – *Life* magazine published a cover story on Wasson's ground-breaking "Seeking the Magic

Mushroom" and Pavlovna's "I Ate the Sacred Mushroom" appeared on the cover of *This Week,* a Sunday magazine inserted in 37 newspapers.

All of a sudden, magic mushrooms were a thing. It was the first time psychoactive mushrooms were introduced to a wide audience – and Wasson is credited with coining the term *magic mushroom.* An unfortunate side effect of all the buzz about these fungi was the start of psychedelic travel, with famous folks (Bob Dylan, Mick Jagger, John Lennon) and regular folks traveling to Mexico in search of Sabina and other healers.

Since the 1950s, psilocybin has been used extensively in clinical research, with more than 40,000 patients receiving this medicine without serious adverse events.

Read more about the benefits and effects of psilocybin in Chapter 3.

" INSPIRING QUOTE "The increased awareness offered by psychedelics comes in different forms. In higher doses taken in safe and sacred settings, they facilitate recognition of one's intimate relationship with all living things. In moderate doses, they facilitate awareness of the intricate psychodynamic structures of one's individual consciousness. In low [micro] doses, they facilitate awareness of solutions to technical and artistic problems." - JAMES FADIMAN **"**

AYAHUASCA: A plant-medicine brew known as the "vine of the soul" is prepared from the combination of the Ayahuasca vine and the leaves of the Chacruna shrub that grows naturally in the Amazon in South America. Also called caapi, yaje, or yage, this DMT-infused "tea" has been used for healing and community for thousands of years, though traditionally, only the shaman (or healers) drank the tea. Numerous Indigenous people use Ayahuasca, but the Shipibo are credited with protecting the sacredness of the medicine – especially after Spanish Jesuit missionaries called out Ayahuasca as the work of the devil and attempted to ban its use.

Interestingly, also in the 1950s, "beat" author and well-known drug user and heroin addict William S. Burroughs went on a journey in 1952 through South America on a quest to find his "final fix." In *The Yage Letters,* he recounts his experiences through letters to fellow beat author Allen Ginsberg.

By the 1960s, Ayahuasca quests were in full effect, with Western tourists traveling to Peru, Columbia, Bolivia, Ecuador, and Brazil seeking healing – and as the decades passed, more and more people have gone on healing quests to South America, some working with shamans while others simply bought the brew from a local vendor.

Earlier this century, neuroscientists finally started researching how Ayahuasca affects the brain.

While Ayahuasca can be found in underground centers in the United States and in limited religious centers, most people still travel to Peru (or Mexico or Costa Rica), where it is legal. The latest statistics show that Iquitos, the town at the center of Ayahuasca and filled with multiple lodges and retreat centers (as well as shamans), brought in almost $7 million from foreign tourists seeking the brew.

Read more about the benefits and effects of Ayahuasca in Chapter 3.

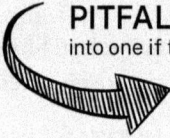

PITFALLS TO HEALING Never rush a psychedelic journey or go into one if things do not feel/seem right. If you're not feeling the medicine, don't do it. There will always be another opportunity to take a psychedelic journey and obtain healing when the set and setting are correct.

MESCALINE: This psychedelic medicine is found in just a handful of cacti and its use can be traced back 6,000 years, to prehistoric peoples participating in ceremonies in the Rio Grande area of Texas. It also has a long history of use by Indigenous peoples in Central and South America.

Mescaline became a "thing" when Aldous Huxley took the medicine for the first time in the 1950s and wrote a series of essays that was then published in book form with the title *The Doors of Perception.*

The two cacti with the highest amounts of mescaline are the San Pedro (also known as *Huachuma)* and peyote cacti, though it is also found in the Peruvian torch, the Bolivian torch, and to an even lesser amount in other species of cacti.

Following the same thinking as with magic mushrooms and Ayahuasca, Catholic priests saw the sacred use of the peyote as the work of the devil and tried to squash the use of mescaline in Mexico, Peru, and the entire region.

In 1897, Arthur Heffter, a German pharmacologist and chemist, extracted mescaline from peyote. His investigations showed that the effects of mescaline can be felt at 100 mg, but 350 mg is needed for a psychotropic experience.

In 1918, the federal government attempted to ban peyote as a narcotic. To protect themselves, the Indigenous tribes in Oklahoma incorporated the Native American Church, to give their sacrament legal status under the First Amendment's freedom of worship.

Read more about the benefits and effects of mescaline in Chapter 3.

LSD: Swiss chemist Albert Hoffman first derived LSD in 1938 from a chemical (lysergic acid) derived from ergot, a fungus that infects grain. However, he did not discover the drug's hallucinogenic effect until five years later when he accidentally ingested a small amount of LSD and saw "extraordinary shapes with intense, kaleidoscopic play of colors."

A few days later, Hoffman intentionally took a larger dose of the drug and rode his bike home – one of the most famous bike rides in history! (Years later, April 19 came to be celebrated by some recreational LSD users as Bicycle Day.) Hoffman's work became a catalyst for other researchers in studying other psychedelics, such as psilocybin and DMT.

LSD-assisted psychotherapy was used in the 1950s and early 1960s by psychiatrists, with very positive results for thousands of patients – and accepted as mainstream therapy tool. During this same period, six international conferences, more than 1,000 scientific papers, and several books were written about the use of LSD in psychiatry.

Because of the Cold War with the then Soviet Union, the Central Intelligence Agency (CIA) got involved in using and testing LSD to see if it could be used in various capacities, such as for mind control, interrogations, and for disarming enemy combatants.

Unfortunately, in the late 1960s, LSD became synonymous with the hippie and anti-war counterculture movement – especially when Dr. Timothy Leary, a psychology professor with Harvard University, became a sort of cult figure in the psychedelics movement. Leary first tried psychedelics on a trip to Mexico, where he ingested psilocybin; he was so impressed that he created the Harvard Psilocybin Project with Richard Alpert (later known as Ram Dass, a colleague at Harvard). Leary later moved on to studying LSD – before getting fired from Harvard for not teaching his classes (because he was so busy evangelizing psychedelics).

By the mid-1960s, Leary began evangelizing about the benefits of LSD and other psychedelics, encouraging celebrities and other to join in… later becoming famous for his classic catchphrase of "turn on, tune in, drop out."

> **INSPIRING QUOTE** "The shadow goes by many familiar names: the disowned self, the lower self, the dark twin or brother in bible and myth, the double, repressed self, alter ego, id. When we come face-to-face with our darker side, we use metaphors to describe these shadow encounters: meeting our demons, wrestling with the devil, descent to the underworld, dark night of the soul, midlife crisis." – CONNIE ZWEIG

Sadly, President Richard Nixon and Congress – perhaps fearful of the growing anti-war movement about the U.S. presence in Vietnam – decided that LSD was a cultural threat to American values, and in 1966 passed the Drug Abuse Control Amendment (which banned the manufacturing or sale of LSD and similar hallucinogens). Four years later, Congress passed the Comprehensive Drug Abuse Prevention and Control Act of 1970, listing LSD (and most other psychedelics) as a Schedule I drug, meaning that it has no medicinal value. Shortly thereafter, the United Nations also established a worldwide ban on psychedelics – and ALL research with LSD evaporated… and disappeared.

Read more about the benefits and effects of LSD in Chapter 3.

MDMA: First developed by scientists at Merck in 1912 when they were looking for a parent compound to synthesize medications that control bleeding.

MDMA, like LSD, was used by some psychiatrists in therapy during the late 1970s and early 1980s – despite that the drug had never undergone any clinical trials nor been approved for human use by the FDA. Psychiatrists found that MDMA was a useful tool in helping patients open up for talk therapy.

MDMA has been described by some as an "empathogenic" drug because of its empathy-producing effects. Results of several studies show the effects of increased empathy with others. When an individual ingests MDMA, three neurotransmitters are released – serotonin, dopamine, and norepinephrine – meaning that there are more "feel-good" chemicals in the brain causing feelings of intense happiness, pleasure, and euphoria.

Also like LSD, MDMA became extremely popular on the streets with the party crowd. MDMA was nicknamed *Molly* and *Ecstasy* – and got the attention of the government, and in 1985, the DEA declared an emergency ban on MDMA, putting it on the list of Schedule I drugs, claiming it had no accepted medical use and a high potential for abuse.

Amazingly, in the early 1990s, Rick Doblin and his non-profit, Multidisciplinary Association for Psychedelic Studies (MAPS), were able to attain FDA approval for MDMA clinical trials. Furthermore, the FDA granted Breakthrough Ther-

PITFALLS TO HEALING It's important to consider using a supplement such as 5-HTP (one of the major ingredients the body needs to make serotonin) to help replace the large amounts of serotonin released by the use of MDMA. The lack of serotonin can cause feelings of deep sadness and depression, a lack of motivation, and feelings of malaise after an MDMA journey.

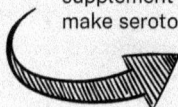

apy designation to MDMA. MAPS is now in third phase trials, examining the use of MDMA in treating post-traumatic stress disorder (PTSD).

Read more about the benefits and effects of MDMA in Chapter 3.

KETAMINE: A more recent discovery, ketamine dates back to 1962 when it was first synthesized by American scientist Calvin Stevens at the Parke Davis Laboratories; it's a medication primarily used for induction and maintenance of anesthesia. It was originally developed as a replacement for PCP. It induces dissociative anesthesia, a trance-like state providing pain relief, sedation, and amnesia – and is considered a hallucinogen – but not a classic psychedelic (such as LSD, psilocybin, mescaline, DMT). As a dissociative, ketamine can make people feel disconnected from their physical bodies.

The FDA approved ketamine as an anesthetic agent in 1970, and it has been used safely in adults, children, pets, and livestock for more than 50 years.

Ketamine was a key tool used in the Vietnam War – as an anesthetic that soldiers could use on the battlefield to help each other rather than waiting for a medic.

In the late 1970s, two key books were published on ketamine: Marcia Moore wrote *Journeys into the Bright World* (an intimate personal story of a husband-wife duo, their love and their explorations into higher consciousness via ketamine) and John Lilly wrote *The Scientist* (an autobiography covering his entire life and science projects, including breakthroughs with consciousness expanding drugs, including ketamine, and isolation tanks, which gave more recognition to the dissociative effects of ketamine).

In the 1990s, ketamine began to be popularly used (and abused) in the club scene – called Special K, Vitamin K, Cat Tranquilizer, and Kit Kat – which is why it is now known as a club drug. When the drug is used recreationally, it can produce out of body experiences, hence the reason that ketamine is referred to as a dissociative anesthesia.

Happily, researchers discovered that ketamine works on glutamate receptors and has antidepressant effects. In some patients with depression who have never responded to anything else, ketamine can lead to a rapid response; it can reduce depressive symptoms within hours.

Read more about the benefits and effects of ketamine in Chapter 3.

IBOGAINE: A naturally-occurring psychoactive substance with dissociative properties found in the roots of shrubs in the family Apocynaceae such as Tabernanthe iboga (as well as Voacanga africana, and Tabernaemontana undulata), and native to the rain forest of central and west Africa. Ibogaine is used by

Indigenous peoples in low doses to combat fatigue, hunger, and thirst, and in higher doses, as a sacrament in religious rituals.

Researchers now understand that Ibogaine rewires the brain, relieves withdrawal symptoms, and gets rid of opioid cravings in just a few hours. The results can last for weeks, months, or sometimes longer.

Ibogaine has been used for centuries by African Indigenous people, and was first observed/reported by French and Belgian explorers in the 19th century.

In the 1930s (and for the next three decades), Ibogaine was sold as tablets (with the brand name Lambarene) in France, with a package insert stating: "a neuromuscular stimulant, promoting cell combustions and getting rid of fatigue, indicated in cases of depression, asthenia, in convalescence, infectious diseases, greater than normal physical or mental efforts by healthy individuals. 2-4 Tablets daily. Rapid and prolonged action, not followed by depression. May be administered to hypertensives."

In 1962, Howard Lotsof became the first person to discover the medical benefits of Ibogaine for the treatment of opiate addiction. Later in the 1960s, Ibogaine was synthesized. In 1969, Claudio Narjano was granted a French patent for the use of Ibogaine in psychotherapy.

As with all the other medicines mentioned in this section, Ibogaine was placed on the list of banned Schedule I drugs in 1967. Ironically, in the 1980s and 1990s, Ibogaine was proven to show positive effects in promoting long-term abstinence from addictive substances – reducing the addiction/dependence to psychostimulants and opiates, including morphine, cocaine, and alcohol. (Other promising psychedelics for drug addiction treatment include LSD and psilocybin from magic mushrooms.)

Read more about the benefits and effects of Ibogaine in Chapter 3.

DMT: Is found naturally-occurring in many plants, animals – **and even people** – and has been used (indirectly) by Indigenous people are centuries. (DMT has been found in 400 kinds of plants and fungi.) The largest percentage of the plants which contain DMT are native to South America. For many years, DMT

INSPIRING QUOTE "Entheogens (or psychedelics, to be more historically correct) have now been recognized as the mother of our Western ecology and conservation movements, as well as the entire field of transpersonal psychology and our apparent desire to return to some firsthand spiritual and/or mystical understanding of God — rather than blindly accepting traditional religious dogma without an experiential basis." – JAMES OROC

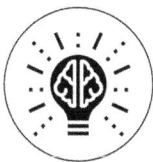

was consumed as part of a plant ceremony; for example, the key element within Ayahuasca is DMT.

Not to be confused with 5-MeO-DMT, which is about 6 times more powerful than DMT, and is a bit more controversial, especially since most is harvested from the venom of the Sonoran Desert Toad. (There's been a slow, but strong push for shifting to the use of synthetic formulations of 5-MeO-DMT.)

DMT's psychoactive properties were first studied scientifically by the Hungarian chemist and psychologist Stephen Szara, who performed research with volunteers in the mid-1950s.

Interestingly, Albert Hofmann, well-known for his synthesis and work with LSD, also synthesized a number of DMT analogs.

Dr. Timothy Leary, along with fellow researchers Richard Alpert and Ralph Metzner, are credited with being key to DMT's many years of popular psychedelic use.

But in more recent years, people are using (smoking) DMT directly because of its potency – DMT is also referred to as the "spirit molecule" due to the intense psychedelic experience it offers and that most people report seeing God, the Creator, and other other-worldly creatures.

Read more about the benefits and effects of DMT in Chapter 3.

U.S. DRUG POLICY

As discussed earlier in this chapter, the "abuses" of LSD in the 1960s and MDMA in the 1980s as party and "hippie" drugs, led to the Federal Government panicking about all psychedelic substances and plants; but decades later, we are seeing a softening of that stance.

Still, we have a long history – decades – for which much of the population has been told by the government that these psychedelic and plant medicines are harmful, addictive, and with no therapeutic use… all false claims.

At the same time, we are now seeing athletes and celebrities coming out and announcing their big psychedelic experiences – or having psychedelic parties.

Many in the psychedelic community are fearful of backlash from the recreational use of these medicines. These ARE medicines and they ARE tools to healing and recovery when the integration work is done. So, we may see more communities and states (and perhaps even at the Federal level) do something – whether it is legalization, decriminalization, or FDA-approval of the medicines – but we may also see that enthusiasm for allowing these medicines to be available to all people being scaled back dramatically.

> **INSPIRING QUOTE** "When we do plant medicine, and we see love, we realize right then and there that it was never apart from us, that in fact it was a part of us."
> – GERARD ARMOND POWELL

KEY TERMS

The *War on Drugs* became a slogan and a mantra when President Richard Nixon and Congress, desperate to hold together the American culture and the War in Vietnam, decided to outlaw all psychedelics by establishing the Controlled Substances Act and putting these clearly therapeutic medicines on the highest schedule level, along with the likes of heroin.

In an interview years later, John Ehrlichman, President Nixon's trusted legal counsel and Assistant to the President for Domestic Affairs, stated: "We knew we couldn't make it illegal to be either against the war or Black, but by getting the public to associate the hippies with marijuana and Blacks with heroin, and then criminalizing both heavily, we could disrupt those communities. We could arrest their leaders, raid their homes, break up their meetings, and vilify them night after night on the evening news. Did we know we were lying about the drugs? Of course we did."

The current list of Schedule I drugs also includes cannabis, bath salts, quaaludes, khat, synthetic cannabis, and GHB. Amazingly, cocaine, amphetamines, and oxycodone – all highly addictive – are on the next level down – Schedule II drugs. Another powerful anti-anxiety drug, Xanax – also highly addictive – is a Schedule IV drug.

Amazingly, more than 50 years after the start of the War on Drugs, including nine different presidents from both political parties, neither Congress nor any president has attempted to end the nonsensical war.

Schedule I Drugs, according to the U.S. Department of Drug Enforcement (DEA), have three conditions:

- *The drug is highly addictive and has a high potential for abuse;*
- *The drug has no currently accepted medical benefits;*
- *The drug has a lack of accepted safety for use under medical supervision.*

Just Say No became a catchphrase came in the 1980s when President Ronald Reagan (and wife Nancy) introduced it as part of an escalation on the War on Drugs – especially because of the escalation of crack and cocaine use in the U.S. *Just Say No* club organizations within schools and school-run anti-drug programs soon became common, with students making pacts not to use recreational drugs.

D.A.R.E. (Drug Abuse Resistance Education) was developed as a curriculum for schools by Dr. Ruth Rich, Health Education Curriculum Administrator for the Los Angeles Unified School District, and emphasized teaching detailed information about specific drugs and their negative effects. In 1984, D.A.R.E. created and implemented a middle-school curriculum. In 1989, D.A.R.E. introduced a high school curriculum. (More recently, D.A.R.E. has expanded its curriculum, also covering alcohol, violence, bullying, and internet safety.)

Legalization is the process of removing all legal prohibitions of a specified substance, including possession, use and manufacturing – at all levels and for any usage.

Decriminalization keeps the medicine illegal, but removes criminal sanctions, so that the legal system will not pursue individual users caught with the drugs, under a certain amount. Under decriminalization, the commercial use/possession is completely illegal, but personal use is allowed.

FDA-approved means the medicines are available only through prescription – and used under a doctor's care – and only for therapeutic use.

KEY LEADERS AND PIONEERS OF THE PSYCHEDELIC MOVEMENT

RICK DOBLIN, Ph.D., best known as the founder and executive director of the nonprofit Multidisciplinary Association for Psychedelic Studies (MAPS), has worked tirelessly for more than 3 decades in promoting the use of psychedelics and cannabis as tools/medicines for healing. He received his doctorate in Public

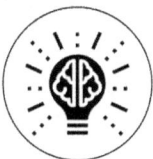

FUN FACT The 2021 Global Drug Survey found that one in four recent users of psychedelics had tried microdosing.

Policy from Harvard's Kennedy School of Government, where he wrote his dissertation on the regulation of the medical uses of psychedelics and marijuana. He also trained with Dr. Stanislav Grof and was among the first to be certified as a Holotropic Breathwork practitioner. His professional goal is to help develop legal contexts for the beneficial uses of psychedelics and marijuana, primarily as prescription medicines but also for personal growth for otherwise healthy people, and eventually to become a legally licensed psychedelic therapist.

JAMES FADIMAN, Ph.D., who has been called "America's wisest and most respected authority on psychedelics and their use," has been involved with psychedelic research since the 1960s when he was introduced to psychedelics for the first time by his friend Richard Alpert (an associate of Timothy Leary, who later became more famously known as Ram Dass) and began his historic role in psychedelic research. Fadiman has also been labeled the "Father of Microdosing" for his pioneering exploration and scientific studies of the use and effects of microdosing. He earned a bachelor's from Harvard and both his master's and doctorate degrees from Stanford, and is a leader in the microdosing of psychedelics movement. He is a published author whose most famous book is *The Psychedelic Explorer's Guide: Safe, Therapeutic, and Sacred Journeys*. He and Robert Frager co-founded the Institute of Transpersonal Psychology, which later became Sofia University (a for-profit, private school), where he is currently a lecturer in psychedelic studies.

ROLAND GRIFFITHS, MD, who is my all-time favorite doctor, though I have only "met" him through numerous documentaries on psychedelics, because of his gentle ways and kind personality – as well as his impactful work with psychedelics. He is a professor of neuroscience, psychiatry, and behavioral science – as well as director of the Center for Psychedelic and Consciousness Research at Johns Hopkins University School of Medicine, one of the premier centers conducting medicinal psychedelic research. Griffiths is credited with reviving interest in clinical trials and research with psychedelic medicines in the late 2000s, examining their potential for treatment of addiction, depression, and anxiety.

> **INSPIRING QUOTE** "No wonder psychedelics are threatening to an authoritarian religious hierarchy. You don't need faith to benefit from a psychedelic experience, let alone a priest or even a shaman to interpret it. What you need is courage—courage to drink the brew, eat the mushroom, or whatever it is, and then to pay attention, and make of it what you will. Suddenly, the tools for direct contact with the transcendent other (whether you call it God or something else) is taken from the hands of an anointed elite and given to the individual seeker." – DENNIS MCKENNA, PH.D.

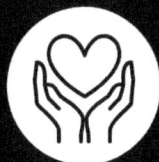

He is an international leader in psychopharmacology research, with a special emphasis on the pharmacology of drugs of abuse. He is the author of more than 400 scientific articles and book chapters and has made significant contributions to our understanding of a wide range of drugs, with a particular focus on sedative-hypnotics, caffeine, and psychedelic substances.

RICK STRASSMAN, MD., a Clinical Associate Professor of Psychiatry at the University of New Mexico School of Medicine, he is best known for being the first person in the United States to restart (ending a 20-year hiatus) human research with psychedelic, hallucinogenic, or entheogenic substances with his work with the powerful naturally-occurring psychedelic compound, DMT (N,N-dimethyltryptamine), during the period 1990-1995. He published a seminal book, *DMT: The Spirit Molecule*, an account of his DMT and psilocybin studies. He co-produced an independent documentary by the same name, which was the most-streamed independent drug documentary on Netflix. He also is the author of *DMT and the Soul of Prophecy*. He has published more than 40 peer-reviewed scientific papers. His most recent book, *The Psychedelic Handbook*, is a great reference for understanding the science and history of psychedelics; and discovering their potential to treat depression, PTSD, substance abuse, and other disorders, as well as to increase wellness, creativity, and meditation.

ALEXANDER "SASHA" SHULGIN, a true legend in the field and dubbed the *godfather of psychedelics*, was an American medicinal chemist, biochemist, organic chemist, pharmacologist, psychopharmacologist, and author. He is best known for his synthesis, creation, and personal bioassay of hundreds of novel psychoactive compounds. After serving in the U.S. Navy during World War II, Sasha earned his Ph.D. in biochemistry from the University of California, Berkeley, and completed post-doctoral work in the fields of psychiatry and pharmacology at the University of California, San Francisco. He worked for Dow, where some of his initial experimenting was done, as well as worked with the DEA. In 1988, he authored the definitive manual *Controlled Substances: Chemical & Legal Guide to Federal Drug Laws* (with an updated second edition appearing in 1992). In order to carry out his research, Sasha obtained a DEA Schedule I license for an analytical laboratory, allowing him to possess and synthesize scheduled substances. He is credited with introducing 3,4-meth-ylenedioxymethamphetamine (MDMA) to psychologists in the late 1970s for psychopharmaceutical use and helping the widespread use of MDMA. He and his second wife Ann (who played a major role in his research and testing) were passionate advocates for the use of psychedelics in therapeutic contexts

ALBERT HOFMANN, Ph.D., a Swiss chemist who worked in the pharmaceutical/chemical department of Sandoz Laboratories, and is best known for being the first to synthesize, ingest, and learn the psychedelic effects of lysergic acid diethylamide (LSD), which he first synthesized in 1938 by isolating compounds found in ergot (*Claviceps purpurea*), a fungus affecting rye. Hofmann's team also isolated, named, and synthesized the principal compounds found within magic mushrooms – psilocybin and psilocin. He authored more than 100 scientific articles and numerous books, including *LSD: Mein Sorgenkind* (*LSD: My Problem Child*). Hofmann's research with LSD influenced several psychiatrists, including Ronald A. Sandison, who developed its use in psychotherapy. Most of Hoffman's later research focused on the psychotropic qualities of various plants and fungi.

STANISLAV GROF, MD, Ph.D., a Czechoslovakia-born psychiatrist with more than 160 academic articles and books, and best known for his early work with LSD and later for his use of breathwork for altering consciousness. Following the suppression of LSD for research in the late 1960s (thanks to it being placed on Schedule I), Grof moved his attention to developing a theory that many states of mind would be explored without drugs by using certain breathing techniques. He postulated that there are two modes of consciousness – hylotropic and holotropic – in which hylotropic mode deals with the "normal, everyday experience of consensus reality" and holotropic mode deals with non-ordinary states of consciousness, such as meditative, mystical, or psychedelic experiences. Dr. Grof is Professor of Psychology at the California Institute of Integral Studies (CIIS) in the Department of Philosophy, Cosmology, and Consciousness in San Francisco. In August 2019, he published his life's work in *The Way of the Psychonaut* – and later appeared in the documentary film about his life and work: *The Way of the Psychonaut - Stan Grof and the Journey of Consciousness.*

PITFALLS TO HEALING While there has been promising evidence of safety and effectiveness for psychedelics after a few acute macrodoses in clinical trials, the risks and benefits of chronic microdosing still remain largely unknown, so do your research as you consider microdosing.

CHARLES GROB, MD, a professor of psychiatry and biobehavioral sciences and pediatrics at the David Geffen School of Medicine at UCLA and director, Division of Child and Adolescent Psychiatry, Harbor-UCLA Medical Center. His research has included the first FDA-approved Phase 1 study of the physiological and psychological effects of MDMA (3,4-methylenedioxymethamphetamine); a multi-national, collaborative study of Ayahuasca in Brazil; and a pilot investigation of the safety and efficacy of psilocybin in the treatment of anxiety in adult patients with advanced-stage cancer. His most recent research has examined the safety and efficacy of an MDMA treatment model with adult autistics with severe social anxiety. Grob is also the editor of *Hallucinogens: A Reader*, originally published in 2002 – a collection of psychedelic texts covering a wide range of topics, such as shamanism, society, and psilocybin research. It contains excerpts from key pioneers of the psychedelic movement, including Terrence McKenna, Albert Hoffman, and Ralph Metzner.

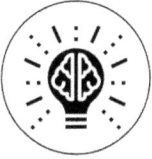

FUN FACT While many interested in mescaline focus on the peyote cactus, the use of the Huachuma cactus, native to the Andres Mountains, can be traced back more than 4,000 years in Peru. The cactus was renamed San Pedro – Saint Peter – because of the belief that users of the cactus can "reach heaven while still on Earth."

RALPH METZNER, Ph.D., psychonaut and pioneering researcher of consciousness, he dedicated his life to teaching and writing about regular and altered states of consciousness. He was researching the therapeutic potential of psilocybin and LSD even before the general public was even aware it existed. In the 1970s, his exploration reoriented toward transformations of consciousness induced by practices such as yoga, meditation, alchemy, and new psychotherapeutic methods using deep altered states. Later on, he became intensely interested in shamanic practices of Indigenous Mesoamerican and Amazonian peoples. Metzner was a psychotherapist and Professor Emeritus of psychology at the California Institute of Integral Studies, based in San Francisco. He was a co-founder and President of the Green Earth Foundation, a nonprofit educational organization devoted to healing and harmonizing the relationship between humans and the Earth. Metzner was featured in the 2006 film *Entheogen: Awakening the Divine Within*, a documentary about rediscovering an enchanted cosmos in the modern world.

TERENCE MCKENNA, often referred to as the "Timothy Leary of the 1990s," he was considered a key pioneer in the field of psychedelics. He admitted that he was heavily influenced by the 1957 *Life* magazine article written by amateur mycologist R. Gordon Wasson, "Seeking the Magic Mushroom." With the help of his brother, Dennis McKenna, who is also a pioneer in the field, Terence developed a new technique for cultivating psilocybin mushrooms. The brothers were the first to create a reliable method for cultivating these types of mushrooms, enabling at-home cultivation of psilocybin mushrooms, publishing their new technique in *Psilocybin: Magic Mushroom Grower's Guide*. He spoke and wrote about a variety of subjects, including psychedelics, plant-based entheogens, shamanism, metaphysics, alchemy, language, philosophy, environmentalism, and the theoretical origins of human consciousness. He preferred plant medicines over chemical ones produced in the lab: "I think drugs should come from the natural world and be use-tested by shamanically orientated cultures ... one cannot predict the long-term effects of a drug produced in a laboratory."

" INSPIRING QUOTE "Mushrooms expand your thought process. They open up new neural pathways in your brain. Alcohol shuts your brain down. It closes it. It puts holes in your fucking brain." – LUKE ROCKHOLD **"**

DENNIS MCKENNA, Ph.D., the other half of the dynamic duo McKenna brothers, is one of the nicest people you could meet, and an American ethnopharmacologist, researcher, lecturer, and author whose professional and personal interests are focused on the interdisciplinary study of ethnopharmacology and natural hallucinogens. He is a founding board member and the director of ethnopharmacology at the Heffter Research Institute, a nonprofit organization concerned with the investigation of the potential therapeutic uses of psychedelic medicines. His research has included the pharmacology, botany, and chemistry of Ayahuasca and oo-koo-hé. He has also conducted extensive ethnobotanical fieldwork in the Peruvian, Colombian, and Brazilian Amazon. McKenna's research led to the development of natural products for the Aveda Corporation, as well as greater awareness of natural products and medicines. He has authored or co-authored more than 50 peer-reviewed scientific papers and written books, including *The Brotherhood of the Screaming Abyss: My Life with Terence McKenna*, and co-author of *The Invisible Landscape* with his brother Terence.

TIMOTHY LEARY, Ph.D., a noted psychology professor and researcher at Harvard who became a lightning rod for the psychedelic counter-culture movement in the 1960s, with his signature line: "Turn on, tune in, drop out." Leary's push for recreational use of psychedelics led to him being called "a hero of American consciousness" by Allen Ginsberg, while then-President Richard Nixon labeled him as "the most dangerous man in America." While at Harvard, Leary worked on the Harvard Psilocybin Project from 1960 to 1962 and tested the therapeutic effects of LSD and psilocybin, which were legal in the U.S. at the time. After being forced to leave Harvard over questions about his research methods, he continued to publicly promote psychedelic drugs and became a well-known public figure. Perhaps his biggest contribution to psychedelics is that he popularized the concept of "set and setting," which we still use today: meaning one's mindset (shortened to "set") and the physical and social environment (the "setting") in which the user has the psychedelic experience.

DAVID E. NICHOLS, Ph.D., one of the world's top experts on psychedelics and psychoactive compounds, having synthesized hundreds of novel psychoactive compounds in his career. His research focuses on serotonin receptors as likely targets for hallucinogenic/psychedelic substances and atypical antipsychotic drugs, and the possible roles that these receptor systems may play in normal cognitive function. His contributions include the synthesis and reporting of escaline, LCZ, 6-APB, 2C-I-NBOMe, and other NBOMe variants, and several others, as well as the coining of the term "entactogen." He is the founding president of the Heffter Research Institute (named after German chemist and pharmacologist Arthur Heffter, who first discovered that mescaline was the active component in the peyote cactus). He is currently an adjunct professor at the UNC Eshelman School of Pharmacy, Chapel Hill, NC.

HONORABLE MENTION: Michael Pollan, Author of *How to Change Your Mind*, as well as the Netflix docuseries by the same name. Credit for bringing the psychedelics movement to the general public. He is the Knight Professor of Science and Environmental Journalism at the UC Berkeley Graduate School of Journalism. Besides psychedelics, he has also written about food, including the seminal *The Omnivore's Dilemma*.

> **INSPIRING QUOTE** "The curious property of psychedelics is that they're anti-addictive."
> – JAMES FADIMAN, PH.D.

RECENT TRENDS IN PSYCHEDELICS

Starting about 2020, mainstream media became more interested in the healing potential of psychedelics and psychedelic plant medicines and psychedelic-assisted therapy. Articles appeared in Rolling Stone, Forbes, The Guardian, The Telegraph, The Financial Times, The Wall Street Journal, New York Times, The Economist, Essence, Huffington Post, Vice, Toronto Star, NBC News, CBS News, CNBC, BBC. In 2018, best-selling author Michael Pollan published a mainstream book about psychedelics: *How to Change Your Mind: What the New Science of Psychedelics Teaches Us About Consciousness, Dying, Addiction, Depression and Transcendence*.

Numerous media also cover psychedelics, plant medicines, cannabis, including: Chacruna Chronicles, Leafly, Lucid News, Merry Jane, Microdose, Psychedelics Today, Psychedelic Press, Psychedelic Spotlight, Psychedelic Times, Third Wave, Truffle Report.

And even within the conventional medical community, there is growing momentum to study psychedelics. More than 20 conferences were held in the U.S. covering the latest developments in psychedelic science and medicine.

MISCONCEPTIONS AND MYTHS ABOUT PSYCHEDELICS

One of the hurdles we face with psychedelics is more than five decades of lies and mistruths from the War on Drugs. Many in the general public still have completely unfounded ideas about psychedelics.

Psychedelics have a stigma, which is ironic, because for centuries psychedelic plants and fungi have been revered as holy and sacred – and only used in religious/spiritual healing ceremonies.

Thus, to help foster education and shed some much-needed light on the subject, this section shares and debunks some common false narratives about psychedelics.

1. PSYCHEDELICS ARE ADDICTIVE. Quite the opposite; psychedelics are NOT considered addictive or habit-forming; there is no development of any physical dependence. In fact, if anything, psychedelics are anti-addictive. These medicines are known to produce positive insights that can help people overcome addictions and help patients break through to the underlying emotional and traumatic challenges that led to addiction in the first place.

Do some people misuse these medicines? Perhaps some small portion of the population, but for most of these substances, it is almost impossible to consume them daily, because they do not affect the same parts of the brain that addictive drugs do.

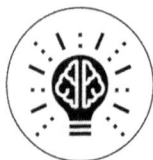

FUN FACT Psychedelics are truly brain medicines – increasing the neuroplasticity of the brain (which aids in new learning and more). Research results from UC Davis: "Our results underscore the therapeutic potential of psychedelics and... on developing plasticity-promoting compounds as safe, effective, and fast-acting treatments for depression and related disorders."

2. PSYCHEDELICS WILL MAKE YOU CRAZY. Remember those public-service ads with the frying pan, "This is your brain on drugs." Ugh. More scare-mongering. On higher doses, will many people hallucinate and see unimaginable visions? Yes, but that's one of the principal properties of psychedelics – and for the vast majority of people, those effects are only temporary until the medicine wears off.

Yes, for people who are already prone to psychosis and mental disorders, psychedelics should NOT be used for concerns about causing a psychotic break.

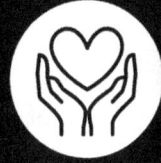

3. PSYCHEDELICS ARE KILLERS. Of EVERY kind of medicine/drug examined over decades and decades of research, psychedelics have been shown to be one of the safest, with the fewest deaths reported. In fact, deaths related to psychedelics are minor compared to deaths from tobacco, alcohol, illicit drugs, and prescription drugs – annually, fewer than 20 deaths are attributed to psychedelic use and more than 700,000 deaths from tobacco, alcohol, illicit drugs, and prescribed medications.

Even at extremely high doses, psychedelics do not lead to physical health problems – even with chronic use. That said, people who take the substances recreationally or ignore the warnings about interactions with other medications, may face health consequences.

4. PSYCHEDELICS ARE PURELY RECREATIONAL. Thousands upon thousands of research studies and papers – both from before the ban on psychedelics in the 1970s and now during this psychedelic renaissance – strongly show the potential for these psychedelic medicines to treat a wide variety of conditions, including: addiction, mood disorders (including depression), anxiety, post-traumatic stress, and control disorders (such as eating disorders, obsessive-compulsive disorder).

Of course, some people will take these medicines recreationally – for the "cool" images and "fun" trip, but even for those people taking these substances recreationally, they are much safer than other recreational drugs such as tobacco and alcohol, let alone heroin, cocaine, etc.

5. PSYCHEDELICS CAN CAUSE BIRTH DEFECTS. This myth has to be the ultimate scare tactic. Psychedelics have NOT been shown to adversely affect sperm, eggs, or DNA. Recent studies have shown that psychedelics do NOT cause any genetic damage nor birth defects.

The question of medicating with psychedelics while trying to get pregnant is more of a personal matter, just like changing diet, supplements, exercise, and other habits while attempting to get pregnant.

It is strongly recommended that women who are pregnant or breast-feeding do not take any psychedelics.

6. PSYCHEDELICS CAN CAUSE HOLES IN THE BRAIN. Have you seen those brain-imaging pictures showing the brain with what looks like big holes in it? Pure propaganda and completely false – except possibly under the most abusive and repeated uses (as with almost any repeated use/abuse of anything).

The truth is that current research shows the opposite of this lie. Psychedelic medicines actually increase the connections in the brain… increase the neuro-plasticity of the brain, making it easier to change your thoughts and behavior in ways that last long-term. Psychedelics may help you make long-term, positive changes to your brain.

7. PSYCHEDELICS WILL RESULT IN REPEATED BAD TRIPS – WITH FLASHBACKS. First, let's state that lower levels/dosages of these medications, including microdosing, do not produce ANY hallucinogenic visions or distortions. Second, let's again rebrand the term "bad trip" to one more applicable – "challenging trip" – because in some instances, people will experience images/visions that are disturbing, frightening, challenging, but these are necessary because the healing comes from uncovering these hidden traumas/fears.

In some situations, certain people (especially it seems from LSD) do have some flashbacks, but the numbers are small and scientists are actively studying why this phenomenon happens to some people. The best news is that these effects are typically temporary.

CHAPTER THREE

Best Practices of Healing Through Psychedelics and
Entheogenic Medicines – Preparation & Integration

In Chapter 2, we learned the history of the major psychedelic medicines, and in this chapter the focus turns to discussing important details about each medicine: how they are currently being used and what to expect during a journey, including duration of effects.

The remainder of this chapter focuses on two critical elements that must be understood and completed to truly have an exceptional journey on the medicine and a fully-optimized life after that journey.

Why do people intentionally consume psychedelics? Typically, for one of three reasons: healing of past traumas (which can manifest as anger, mood disorders, anxiety, addiction, and control disorders); seeking spiritual connection or renewal; inspiring creativity and transformation.

One of the common points made again and again with psychedelics is their power to cut to the core of the problem – of the trauma. Psychedelic medicines facilitate deep breakthroughs that can take months or years to achieve through traditional talk therapy. Very common reactions are along this line: "I achieved in one night what I had not gained in the past five years of therapy." ·

There's also growing evidence about the power of psychedelics to positively influence brain function – that psychedelics can help to boost brain neuroplasti-

FACILITATOR TIP Because there are very limited supplies of peyote left in the Texas/Mexico border region, many people want the Indigenous people to use the peyote for their own ceremonies and for non-Indigenous people to use either synthetic mescaline or mescaline from the San Pedro or other cacti besides peyote.

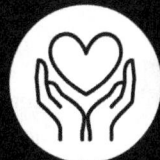

city, making the brain more flexible, potentially helping us learn new behaviors and adapt and make positive changes in our lives. It's possible that increasing neuroplasticity could help break old habits and form new, healthier patterns of behavior. There's also evidence that increased neuroplasticity may help treat depressive symptoms and anxiety.

A PRIMER ON PSYCHEDELICS

PSILOCYBIN – /3-(2-Dimethylaminoethyl)-1H-indol-4-yl/ dihydrogen phosphate – the ingredient in *Magic Mushrooms* (of which there are many varieties). You can harvest and dry the mushrooms themselves or find them online in powder, capsule, and chocolate products. Effects last about 4-5 hours. Psilocybin has a playful element, but its main effect is in freeing the brain from its rigid patterns and allowing users to look at the world and themselves with a new perspective, along with waves of good feelings. Journeys are very inward. Users experience altered psychological functioning in the form of "hypnagogic experiences," which is the transitory state between wakefulness and sleep, and brain imaging studies show that a psilocybin trip is neurologically similar to dreaming. Expect some physical discomfort and varying effects, depending on dosage: low (.5-1.5 grams), medium (1.5-3 grams), high (3-5 grams), and heroic (5+ grams). (https://getheally.com/patients/news/dosing-guide-to-psilocybin) The whole journey lasts about 4-6 hours: The medicine takes about 15-20 minutes to begin; another 30 minutes for the ramp up; peaking for 1-3 hours; coming down for another 2-4 hours. (With heroic or secondary dosages, the journey can last longer.)

66 **INSPIRING QUOTE** "Although many of us think of psychedelics as dangerous drugs, it's time for a rethink. They are non-toxic, non-addictive, have very few side effects, and could potentially offer relief for people suffering from a range of psychological difficulties." – ROSALIND WATTS, PH.D. **99**

AYAHUASCA – a psychoactive brew (with DMT) developed by Indigenous tribes in South America, produced from parts of the Psychotria viridis shrub and Banisteriopsis caapi vine. Effects last about 5-7 hours. Ayahuasca most definitely has a female spirit, which is why many refer to it as Mother Aya. Ayahuasca is very heart-opening and will take you on deep and powerful journeys, but it also sometimes opens a dark/evil shadow side. Typically, people participate in ceremonies with a healer (referred to as shamans when done with Indigenous people) and a small circle of participants. Dosage is controlled by the facilitator/healer, but some people also use Ayahuasca by themselves – not part of a community. Be prepared to purge in some way with Ayahuasca; most commonly

PITFALLS TO HEALING We need to find a way to make psychedelic healing available to everyone. While Black, Indigenous, and people of color (BIPOC) experience similar rates (or greater) of mental health issues as Caucasians, they are greatly underrepresented in clinical research and often lack access to these therapies.

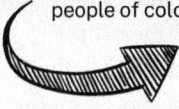

vomiting, but also coughing, laughing, crying, sweating, shaking, and unexpected defecation. Ayahuasca seems to be effective in the treatment of depression and addiction, and PTSD. The whole journey lasts about 5-7 hours: The medicine takes about 20-30 minutes to begin; another 30 minutes for the ramp up; peaking for 2-3 hours; coming down for another 1-3 hours. (With heroic or secondary dosages, the journey can last longer.)

MESCALINE – 3,4,5-trimethoxyphenethylamine – is a naturally-occurring psychedelic protoalkaloid found in some cacti native to the southwest United States, Mexico, and South America, including the peyote cactus, the San Pedro cactus, and the Peruvian Torch cactus. Effects last about 10-12 hours. Most users report a positive experience on mescaline (meaning fewer "bad trips") – the core mescaline effect is a heightened sense of emotional and mental flow. Mescaline is highly hallucinogenic and lends itself to self-exploration; it also creates a uniquely empathic effect in the user, making it useful for personal healing. It's been used to treat depression and post-traumatic stress. Its effects are similar to psilocybin and LSD. Colors become more intense. There is a profound sense of "being in the now," along with a noticeable reduction in mental chatter. People feel euphoric, a sense of one with the world, increased awareness, more energetic, and time distortion. A typical range for starting mescaline hydrochloride (HCl) is 200-300 mg. Anywhere between 300-500 mg is considered strong, while 500-700+ mg is considered a heavy dose. The whole journey lasts about 8-14 hours: The medicine takes about 30-90 minutes to begin; another 60-90 minutes for the ramp up; peaking for 4-6 hours; coming down for another 2-3 hours. (With heroic or secondary dosages, the journey can last longer.)

LSD – Lysergic acid diethylamide – a synthetic chemical made from a substance found in ergot (a fungus that infects rye). The onset of a journey is about 30 minutes, and the whole experience lasts about 10-12 hours. There are numerous strains/types of LSD, each with slightly different reactions/trips, so conduct your research on your supplier. There may soon be more clinical trials using LSD to treat any number of conditions, including: depression, anxiety, PTSD, OCD, and addiction. Effects are generally pleasant, with intensified visual and auditory distortions (including a sharpened sense of taste, smell, hearing), feelings of euphoria and connection, tingling sensation in the skin, and the emergence of new insights and inspiration. LSD works in VERY low dosages: standard dose (strong shift in perception, new ideas) in the 80-200 micrograms range; heroic dose (dramatic shifts in perception, thinking) in the 200-400 microgram range. The whole journey lasts about 8-12 hours: The medicine takes about 20-40 minutes to begin; another 45-90 minutes for the ramp up; peaking for 3-5 hours; coming down for another 3-5 hours. (With heroic or secondary dosages, the journey can last longer.)

FACILITATOR TIP Microdosing to gain trust and get to know the medicine before a future macrodose is a growing trend for why some people are turning to micro-dosing psychedelics.

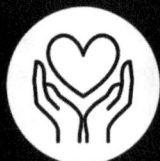

MDMA – 3,4-methylenedioxymethamphetamine – a synthetic chemical that acts as both a stimulant and psychedelic, producing an energizing effect, distortions in time and perception, and enhanced enjoyment of tactile experiences. Extremely heart-opening and external; great for talking/sharing. About 30- 60 minutes after taking the drug, the characteristic effects (euphoria, increased empathy and energy, enhanced sensations) come on and typically last for 3-5 hours; this state is characterized by a sense of relaxation, including emotional openness, reduction of negative thoughts, and a decrease in inhibitions. MDMA can make users feel like all is well in the world, and connecting with others becomes easy. Bodily sensations and touch become enhanced, and sounds and colors can appear more intense. MDMA increases the activity of three brain chemicals: dopamine (increases energy), norepinephrine (increases heart rate and blood pressure), and serotonin (elevates mood and empathy; affects appetite and sleep). Effects last about 4-6 hours, although many users take a second "booster" dose as the effects of the first dose begin to fade, increasing the length to 6-8 hours. If you have secured real MDMA (warning: a lot of "street" MDMA is not MDMA at all), you can maximize the most desirable effects and minimize undesirable effects at doses between 81-100 mg. Another way to examine it is no more than your weight in kg, plus 50 = total dosage in milligrams for the session – not to exceed 120 mg. The whole journey lasts about 4-6 hours: The medicine takes about 30-60 minutes to begin; another 15-30 minutes for the ramp up; peaking for 90-150 minutes; coming down for another 1-2 hours. (With heroic or secondary dosages, the journey can last longer.)

KETAMINE – (±)-2-(2-Chlorophenyl)-2-(methylamino)cyclohexanone – is labeled as a dissociative and was developed as an anesthesia for surgery, but in subanesthetic doses, it induces profound psychedelic experiences, hallucinations, and detachment from both the environment and self. Users may experience numbness, a tingling body high (especially in the hands, feet, and head), jerky movements, rapid breathing, and dizziness; these effects are often accompanied by euphoria, relaxation, a feeling of weightlessness, mild visuals, and blurred or roving vision. Similar to psilocybin, users may also experience introspective thoughts and enhanced appreciation for music. Unlike classical psychedelics (such as LSD and psilocybin), ketamine acts on the brain's glutamate systems and NMDA receptors – and while it's not known exactly how ketamine works, experts believe the drug may repair damaged synapses—or connections–in the brain, which are worn down by stress and depression. Ketamine is being used for depression and other mood disorders, anxiety, OCD, PTSD, and certain addictions/substance use disorders. Effects last about 20 minutes to 1 hour. Ketamine treatment is available at FDA-approved treatment centers around the country (usually by IV), as well as through several online centers (typically in pill form). Dosage is calculated by milligrams of ketamine per kilogram (or pound) of a person's body mass and expressed as mg/kg; for most situations, the recommendation is a dosage of 0.5mg per kg – so, for example, if a person weighs 60kg, the calculation is as follows: 0.5 × 60 = 30mg of ketamine. A nasal spray form of the drug, called esketamine, has also been approved by the Food and Drug Administration for the treatment of major depression. The whole journey lasts about 60-90 minutes: The medicine takes about 2-5 minutes to begin; another 5-10 minutes for the ramp up; peaking for 30-60 minutes; coming down for another 1-2 hours. (With heroic or secondary dosages, the journey can last longer.)

IBOGAINE – 12-Methoxyibogamine – this naturally-occurring substance is a psychedelic with dissociative properties, which has been shown to be especially effective for opioid addiction, and should really only be taken in treatment centers. It stimulates what have been described as "oneirogenic" effects, meaning that it generates a waking dream state. Ibogaine is usually administered in capsule form, depending on the bodyweight of the patient – the effective dose for the treatment of chemical dependence, including opioid dependence, is between 15- 20 mg of Ibogaine per kg. Users can expect to be in bed for the first

FACILITATOR TIP Expect some physical responses to psychedelics as well. Almost all psychedelics have one or more of these physical effects: jaw clenching, trouble regulating body temperature, increased heart rate, lack of sleep, restless limbs, increased respiratory rate, general nausea.

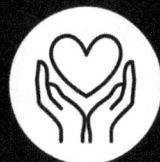

12 hours of the trip (phases 1 and 2). The first several hours will be intense before you start to come down as your body metabolizes the Ibogaine. Typically, users start with a microdose first before taking the macrodose. Users can expect three stages: in the first acute phase, nausea and possible vomiting as well as being sensitive to motion; the skin tends to become numb and many users report an initial buzzing or oscillating sound. In the second, labeled the introspective/reflective stage, users feel a sensation of negative thoughts and emotions being released. In the third, users begin to feel relaxed and positive, often mixed with headaches and body aches. Note: Iboga is dangerous in combination with many substances, so do your due diligence. The whole journey lasts about 36-48 hours: The medicine takes about 45-180 minutes to begin; another 60-90 minutes for the ramp up; peaking for 18-24 hours; coming down for another 24-70 hours. (With heroic or secondary dosages, the journey can last longer.)

DMT – N, N-dimethyltryptamine – the "spirit molecule" is a hallucinogenic that is both a derivative and a structural analog of tryptamine. Interestingly, DMT is produced endogenously (naturally in the body, in the pineal gland in the brain). DMT is the psychoactive ingredient in Ayahuasca, but can also be isolated to pure DMT. Experiences are extreme, but brief: its effects last about 45 minutes when smoked. People ingest DMT in crystal form, smoke it in a pipe or bong, or vaporize it. Higher doses typically produce rapid images full of intensely colorful abstract and representational displays. Auditory hallucinations are less common. Some people experience alternating sensations of hot and cold. Out-of-body experiences, or dissociation of awareness from the physical body, is very common with DMT at higher doses. Many people consider this a hallmark of the experience. In the *DMT: The Spirit Molecule,* Dr. Rick Strassman states that many participants had a "DMT trip or psychological planes where intelligent beings, entities, aliens, guides, and helpers were found." The whole journey lasts about 10-30 minutes: The medicine takes about 20-40 seconds to begin; another 1-3 minutes for the ramp up; peaking for 4-8 minutes; coming down for another 2-6 minutes. (With heroic or secondary dosages, the journey can last longer.)

INSPIRING QUOTE "The visions were not blurred or uncertain. They were sharply focused, the lines and colors being so sharp that they seemed more real to me than anything I had ever seen with my own eyes. I felt that I was now seeing plain, whereas ordinary vision gives us an imperfect view; I was seeing the archetypes, the Platonic ideas, that underlie the imperfect images of everyday life... These reflections passed through my mind at the very time that I was seeing the visions, for the effect of the mushrooms is to bring about a fission of the spirit, a split in the person, a kind of schizophrenia, with the rational side continuing to reason and to observe the sensations that the other side is enjoying." - R. GORDON WASSON

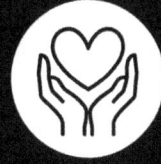

WHAT TO EXPECT FROM A PSYCHEDELIC JOURNEY

While each medicine has its unique characteristics, there are some general physical and psychological effects from medium to higher doses of these medicines.

POSSIBLE PHYSICAL EFFECTS

- *Increased heart rate*
- *Muscle relaxation*
- *Shakes/tremors*
- *Jitteriness*
- *Cramps*
- *Nausea*
- *Vomiting*
- *Pupil dilation*
- *Dry mouth*
- *Sweating*
- *Chills*
- *Numbness*
- *Drowsiness*
- *Sense of body floating (even leaving body – at higher doses)*
- *Sensations related to past diseases, operations, broken bones you've had*

POSSIBLE PSYCHOLOGICAL EFFECTS

- *Heightened awareness of physiological processes (e.g. heartbeat, breathing)*
- *Heightened senses (especially sounds)*
- *Synesthesia (e.g. seeing sounds or hearing colors)*
- *Restlessness*
- *Trouble focusing*
- *Disorientation*
- *Tension*
- *Anxiety*
- *Paranoia*

- *Panic*
- *Euphoria*
- *Visual illusions with eyes open and closed (very high doses)*
- *Intensification of colors*
- *Proprioceptive changes (e.g. body may feel large or tiny)*
- *Experience of merging with the environment/universe*
- *Time and/or space may be experienced as infinite or nonexistent*
- *Highly symbolic experiences (e.g. involving religious or mythical signs, symbols, and scenes, perhaps beyond your own personal field of experience or knowledge)*
- *Perception that the experience will never end*
- *Experiences described as mystical or spiritual in nature*
- *Loss of subjective self-identity, or 'ego dissolution' (very high doses)*
- *Perception of losing your mind or going crazy (related to the 'ego dissolution' experience)*
- *Regression to a younger age*
- *Reliving of the birth experience*

" INSPIRING QUOTE "In my mind, MDMA is a mild drug. People who prefer it to the typical psychedelics tend not to do well when stressed, either by life or by taking more potent mind-bending drugs. MDMA is what I like to call a 'love and light' drug, one that accentuates the positive and minimizes the negative. If only life were so simple." - RICK STRASSMAN, MD. **"**

THE CAUSES OF SUFFERING AND THE NEED FOR PSYCHEDELICS

These psychedelic medicines do an amazing job of shining a bright light on the things that need healing within us. According to Carl Jung (and many others), we all have a shadow side – a dark side – of ourselves.

The shadow side is composed of hidden aspects of our personalities that are deemed unacceptable by society, typically related to shame and trauma. For true health and healing, people need to embrace and integrate the shadow into the whole personality – otherwise it can grow stronger, enhancing the ego.

Some of the causes of our suffering and isolation include:

- *Living in the past… or the future*
- *Choosing fear(s)*
- *Clinging to a (hurt, wrong, false) identity*
- *Disconnection with the world*
- *Death (or living with death)*

- *Being a victim; playing the victim*
- *Addictions and attachments to things that only bring temporary relief*
- *Comparison syndrome*
- *Living a divided life (wearing multiple masks)*
- *Loss of connection to the Divine*

CURRENT RESEARCH ON THE POTENTIAL APPLICATIONS OF PSYCHEDELIC MEDICINES FOR MENTAL HEALTH

While research is ongoing, this is a quick list of the conditions for which early analysis of evidence illustrates psychedelic medicines show great promise as novel and breakthrough therapies:

- *Depression: MDMA, psilocybin, LSD, ketamine, mescaline*
- *Anxiety: MDMA, psilocybin, LSD, ketamine, mescaline*
- *Post-traumatic Stress: MDMA, Ayahuasca, ketamine, psilocybin*
- *Obsessive Compulsive Disorder (OCD): psilocybin, ketamine*
- *Eating Disorders: MDMA, Ayahuasca, ketamine, psilocybin*
- *Substance Use Disorder/Addiction: MDMA, ketamine, Ibogaine, LSD, Ayahuasca, mescaline, psilocybin*
- *Suicidal Ideation: ketamine, mescaline*
- *Cluster headaches/migraines: LSD, microdosing psilocybin, LSD, DMT*
- *Attention Deficit Disorder (ADHD): microdosing LSD, psilocybin*

POSITIVE EXPERIENCES FROM PSYCHEDELIC MEDICINES

Beyond the aforementioned therapeutic effects, many participants report lasting benefits from psychedelic medicines, including:

- *Improved self-esteem*
- *Enhanced mood*
- *Deepened spirituality, divinity*
- *Greater positivity*
- *Stronger sense of connectedness*
- *Heightened optimism*
- *Enriched world view*
- *Mindfulness (and a calmer mind)*
- *Psychological flexibility*

PITFALLS TO HEALING There's a shadow/dark side to Ayahuasca that can lead to negative/scary experiences. Be certain to complete your due diligence if you decide to find a healing center and drink the brew. Mother/Grandmother Aya, as the spirit is called, is usually associated with love and healing, but the wrong shaman/facilitator can turn that love inside out.

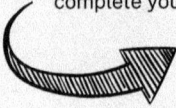

HARM REDUCTION WITH PSYCHEDELICS

Whether you decide on taking these psychedelic medicines at home, in a clinic, or a healing center, harm reduction is a critical factor to address. This is a proactive strategy that aims to minimize any potential negative effects that may occur during psychedelic use/therapy; it should prioritize education, safety, and compassion.

Harm reduction deals with approaches to reduce the harm associated with psychedelic medicine use – not only for the person taking the medicine, but for all others involved. When people are under the influence of a psychedelic, they are extremely vulnerable, and the experience can be overwhelming and disorienting. It is essential to have people (facilitators, trip-sitters, healers) who understand this issue and are who are prepared/trained to offer assistance.

As you do your research for your psychedelic experience, please take the time to be certain that the therapist, clinic, healing center, or tripsitter follow harm reduction practices. Every element of your psychedelic experience – from the initial consultation through the journey and including your integration – should follow harm reduction procedures.

TIPS FOR NAVIGATING A CHALLENGING ("BAD TRIP") JOURNEY

Worried about what some inaccurately call a "bad trip?" This is experiencing challenging situations during your psychedelic journey. These challenging situations are something akin to a nightmare. However, these experiences are intended to be reframed as difficult things needed to be seen in order to move past the trauma and onto healing – resulting in a better life.

Regardless of anything else, please remember that these medicines work best when you use them with intention. Recreational use (aka lack of intention) will not give you the healing results you seek.

1. UNDERSTAND THE RISKS. The first step should always be a risk assessment. Are you physically healthy enough to take psychedelics? Are you mentally prepared for a psychedelic journey? Are you filled with doubts or dread? Are you prepared to surrender to the medicine?

2. DO YOUR RESEARCH ON THE MEDICINE. As you have read in earlier sections of this book, each medicine has its own characteristics, effects, and duration. Obviously, dosage also plays a major role – so know the exact dosage of the medicine that you plan to consume. Review the stories later in the book that describe people's experiences with the medicine.

3. CONFIRM THE MEDICINE YOU ARE CONSUMING. If you are sourcing the medicine from underground sources (the dark web) … First, you need to be aware there are many scammers out there taking advantage of the psychedelic renaissance. Second, you have to ensure that the medicine you received is actually the medicine – and at the correct dosage you seek. Many psychedelics can be tested using kits purchased at sites such as BunkPolice.com or DanceSafe.org.

4. CLEAR AND PREPARE YOUR MIND. On the day of your journey (and ideally for at least a week prior), avoid all stressful situations and take time before the journey to settle yourself, calm your mind, and set up a positive intention for the experience. Meditate, pray, breathe, and relax before starting your journey.

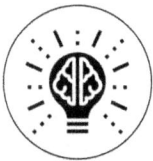

FUN FACT Your dreams may be especially strange and potent both right before and right after a psychedelic trip, so it's important to journal about whatever themes are bubbling up from your unconscious mind.

5. CONFIRM THAT THE SETTING IS SAFE. For me, the best setting for a psychedelic journey is one that is cozy and comfortable. I want all the creature comforts around me, including soft pillows and blankets, pretty surroundings (bright room or out in nature); music; and hydration. Some people also include photos and favorite knick-knacks.

6. GET THE MUSIC RIGHT. Music can play a major role in the psychedelic experience, especially with psilocybin, where music is extremely enhanced, and ketamine, which can alter auditory sensation. Everyone has their own opinions about the type of music that works best – but my suggestion is to choose music you love and that does not have any negative triggers. Some journeyers prefer music with no lyrics at all; some people prefer complete silence or only the sounds of nature. (Definitely avoid angry rap and head-banging music!)

7. SURRENDER, SURRENDER, SURRENDER. It may take some practice, but perhaps the biggest tip for having a good and successful journey involves getting your brain to stop trying to control the experience. It's vital that you not fight the medicine's visions/effects. Some of these elements may be disturbing, but they are temporary – and essential to healing. Again, during a journey, when in doubt… surrender!

8. IF YOU'RE FEELING UNCOMFORTABLE, SEEK ASSISTANCE. One of the great benefits of consuming these medicines in a healing center is there are people there to assist you if you feel you are struggling in your journey. Having a sober partner or tripsitter with you if you are doing your journey by yourself is also a wise choice. Finally, you should have the Fireside Project (623-473-7433) in your phone contacts. (You can also download the Fireside Project app.)

9. STAY HYDRATED. Depending on what medicine you use – and its duration – you will want to keep hydrated throughout your journey. Drink moderately; just water or water with electrolytes.

10. EMBRACE AND ACCEPT. All psychedelic journeys have a flow – from ramp up, to extreme experiences, to ramp down. The best mindset you can have is simply enjoy the ride! It may be a bit difficult, but as you are nearing the start of your journey, let go of all your expectations and clear your mind for what the medicine shows you.

WHAT TO EXPECT FROM A PSYCHEDELIC EXPERIENCE

So… you're seriously considering a psychedelic experience and you're a bit trepidatious and unsure what to expect, right?

Almost ALL the research I have completed over the last several years has given me tremendous insights into the various psychedelic medicines – and yet, there is very little on prepping people for what to expect… which is the driving focus of this book.

While each psychedelic medicine acts differently and has different phases and duration, there are some common elements you can expect from ANY psychedelic experience. That's what this section is about.

" **INSPIRING QUOTE** "It may be that DMT makes us able to perceive what the physicists call 'dark matter' – the 95 percent of the universe's mass that is known to exist but that at present remains invisible to our sense and instruments." – GRAHAM HANCOCK **"**

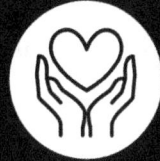

1. INEFFABILITY

Most people who complete psychedelic journeys have an extremely difficult time expressing the details, of putting the experience into words. What you experience – the sights, sounds, visions, feelings – is often difficult to describe to others.

That said, ineffability is one of the reasons why it is so important to start journaling after your psychedelic experience… while still difficult to adequately describe, putting things to paper immediately after your journey is essential.

Ineffability is also why it's so rewarding to share the stories described in the following chapters – and for us all to be very grateful to all these people willing and able to share their experiences.

2. NOVEL EXPERIENCES/INSIGHTS

Reality often takes a major break while you are deep in a psychedelic journey.

Expect to see, feel, hear, experience things like never before. You may also experience new and novel connections and revelations. You may taste the music and hear inanimate objects talking. You may experience out-of-body feelings – from simply floating above your body to traveling to distant and otherworldly planes of existence. The key is to stay open to everything you experience – and to surrender to the experience. (We'll talk more about surrendering in the next section of this chapter.)

Every psychedelic journey is different. Some people see geometric patterns, beautiful colors, energy flows, while others see genies, dead relatives, and crazy distortions of reality. Still others experience few visuals, but have profound new insights. Just be prepared for all types of novel experiences.

3. EGO DEATH/DISSOLUTION

On higher doses (typically on what we call "heroic" doses), something amazing can happen – which is often referred to as ego death or ego dissolution. Ego death is not a death at all (though sometimes it can feel a bit like it) – but a rebirth of the mind and soul into a new way of thinking and living.

Ego death typically only happens during a heavily-dosed psychedelic trip. It is the blurring of the boundaries between the sense of self and the external world, which is why some prefer the somewhat lighter term ego dissolution. It's a temporary loss of – and freedom from – self-identity.

Our sense of reality, perceptions, and views of the world rapidly change – a temporary distortion. Those views are replaced with an overwhelming sense of interconnection with others, with the universe, with the Creator. Joy, unity, and depersonalization temporarily replace our self-centered worldview.

Ego death does not happen all the time and often depends on several factors, including the environment and dosage of the drug. Some people experiencing ego death become anxious and experience a challenging trip. Yet, for many, it's a major leap in consciousness – and a giant step forward in how we see the world and our place in that world. Our goal is to become more aware of the ego and to challenge its (our) stalwart beliefs.

PITFALLS TO HEALING Most people who participate in higher-dosage psychedelic journeys experience ego death, but in a handful of people, instead of the ego dissolving and seeing how tiny we are in this vast universe, their ego expands dramatically. It's part of the "shadow side" of psychedelics and ourselves. This condition can lead to people thinking they should become healers/ shamen… or other grandiose ideas.

4. TIMELESSNESS

Expect to lose track of time during your psychedelic journey.

In fact, put your phone aside and don't even bother with clocks.

In a weird way, time will only exist in your journey – and it will be distorted. Obviously, with short journeys (as with DMT) and extremely long journeys (such as with LSD), you will have fewer issues with time.

The key is to not worry about time and be present IN the journey.

5. HIGHER-ORDER REALITY

Psychedelics raise your level of consciousness, therefore your reality is also going to change with it.

Especially with consuming higher dosages (but it can happen on beginning doses as well) you will get a sense of truly understanding reality – of how the world works, how you fit in it, and what you need to do with this new sense of higher-order reality.

While it seems funny at times hearing stories of flying dragons or aliens or diving deeply into the ocean, the truth is that while on a journey, your reality is truly what you are experiencing.

Furthermore, expect to have one or more grand insights into your world *after* your psychedelic journey, as you begin to integrate all that you experienced.

6. OBSERVER PERSPECTIVE

One of the coolest phenomena of psychedelics is the ability to see yourself, your past, and past traumas in a safe, nonjudgmental environment – as though you are simply observing your past. Make note of what you see and feel.

This detachment from your deep hurts and losses allows you to view these experiences from another perspective. It is this perspective that helps include the novel insights, emotions, or understandings that can arise in psychedelic experiences.

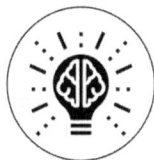

FUN FACT Roughly 10 years after the glowing cover story about R. Gordon Wasson's discovery of magic mushrooms, Life magazine ran an anti-psychedelics cover story in 1966, with the headline: "The Exploding Threat of the Mind Drug That Got Out of Control: LSD." That's how much had changed in politics and culture in that short window of time.

THE FIVE LEVELS OF PSYCHEDELIC EXPERIENCES

Dr. Timothy Leary deconstructed the psychedelic experience into five categories. The five levels of the psychedelic experience range from the very mild – a few random sensations and a sense of well-being – to the extreme, with a complete break with reality and intense hallucinations.

Obviously, every person's experiences with psychedelics are different, but here's a rough idea of what to expect.

LEVEL 1: Light synesthesia (a perceptual phenomenon where sensory and cognitive pathways mingle) and heightened senses, especially with music. Some changes in how you see the world, but the world hasn't changed. Enhanced mood and sensuality.

    MEDICINE: Medium doses of cannabis. Low doses of psilocybin, mescaline, LSD.

LEVEL 2: Minor psychedelic experiences, some visual effects (colors, patterns) and warping of surroundings, as well as some minor closed eye visuals (CEVs). Emotions heightened. Abstract thoughts and unconscious emotions bubble to the surface.

MEDICINE: High doses of cannabis. Low-Medium doses of psilocybin, mescaline. Medium doses of MDMA.

LEVEL 3: True psychedelic experiences, filled with strong visual hallucinations and kaleidoscopic imagery, profound realizations about oneself and the universe, and the slipping away of reality – with some dissociative experiences. High sensitivity to surroundings. Light and sound sensitive.

MEDICINE: Medium doses of psilocybin, mescaline, LSD

LEVEL 4: Deep psychedelic journeys, filled with a departure from reality into new realms – concluding with new and deep changes to self and perception of the world. Expect powerful, otherworld visuals and visions, dissolution of time and reality, out-of-body experiences, and profound realizations. Possible ego dissolution.

MEDICINE: High doses of psilocybin, mescaline, LSD

LEVEL 5: Travel to new realities, with insights from which you will not be the same person. In most cases, people experience ego death/dissolution. There's a total eradication of reality and often the journey includes communications with otherworldly beings. Some sense of traveling at high rates of speeds and being propelled into space. Relatively no difference with what you see – whether your eyes are open or closed. A sense of profound enlightenment with the universe.

MEDICINE: Ayahuasca, DMT, and extremely heroic doses of psilocybin, mescaline, LSD.

66 **INSPIRING QUOTE** "I first explored mescaline in the late '50s... 350 to 400 milligrams. I learned there was a great deal inside me." – ALEXANDER SHULGIN 99

FACTORS INFLUENCING YOUR PSYCHEDELIC EXPERIENCE

One of the great concerns by many people considering psychedelic medicine is the fear of a bad trip, but even that label is misleading, as people sometimes face challenging images and feelings, but rarely is it "bad;" in reality, it is a hallmark of an unattended trauma or problem demanding reconciliation.

That said, there are a few factors that can affect whether your first journey is a good one – or more challenging, including:

- *The psychedelic medicine you ingest*
- *The dosage of the medicine you ingest*
- *The amount of preparation you have completed (see next section)*

- *The set and setting for your journey*
- *The trust you have for the people you are with*
- *The attitude you have for healing your trauma*

PREPARING FOR PSYCHEDELICS: KEYS TO SUCCESS

Depending on the medicine and the setting, your dosage will either be controlled by you or a facilitator. For your first experience, it's best to start on the lower dosing end to see how you will handle the effects. Once you have experienced your first journey, you can decide how to handle the dosage of future experiences.

PREPARATION/DIET

Some experts say you can simply "do" a psychedelic experience, but it's best and more personally rewarding if you prepare for the journey – both mentally and physically.

Regardless of the medicine used, people should make a plan to restrict certain foods, people, and experiences (such as exposure to traditional and social media) at least a week prior to the ceremony – and, ideally, for several weeks prior.

Diet – it's best to eat cleanly – which means eliminating fast foods, processed foods, fried foods, sugar, salt, heavy creams/sauces, and most meats. Eat lots of fresh fruits and vegetables, nuts and grains, and some limited pasture-raised eggs, wild-caught fish, and farm-raised chicken. Consume organic and sustainably-raised foods and meats – not factory foods. Eliminate alcohol, cannabis, recreational drugs.

People – take a break from toxic people in your life; focus on relationships with loved ones and others who truly matter to you.

Experiences – remove yourself from negative situations, discussions, etc. Again, focus your time and energy on positive things, such as creative endeavors and self-improvement.

Screen Time – take a break from social media, news sites, and any other distractions and potentially negative encounters.

" **INSPIRING QUOTE** "LSD is a psychedelic drug which occasionally causes psychotic behavior in people who have NOT taken it." – TIMOTHY LEARY, PH.D. "

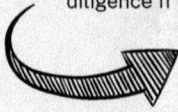

PITFALLS TO HEALING Some antidepressant medications can have dangerous or undesirable interactions with psilocybin, so do your due diligence if taking an antidepressant – and in many cases, you may need to taper down the dosage to get the maximum benefits from the psychedelic medicine. Read more in this post: https://www.psychedelicpassage.com/psilocybin-blunting-effects-of-ssris-and-antidepressants/

SET & SETTING

This section refers to two important aspects of your journey.

Set refers to mindset – what you want to accomplish with the medicine – your intentions. Yes, one can ingest any of these medicines for recreational purposes, for the fun of seeing crazy colors and geometric patterns, but the real work comes from taking the medicine seriously, and you do so by setting an intention.

Your goal is to develop a mindset that believes the psychedelic medicine you ingest will help you see and unlock lost/hidden past traumas – and that it will show you what needs healing/fixing. (Your mindset could also be related to spirituality or transformation.)

An intention is an aspect of what you would like to learn from the medicine – or healing you want from the medicine. An intention helps you stay focused on a goal, even though the medicine may lead you down a completely different path. Your intention should be something easy to remember so it can serve as a mantra for you as you start your journey.

Some examples of intentions:

- *Show me what I am afraid to see about myself*
- *Help me become a more loving person to myself and others*
- *Help me process the trauma from being abused*
- *Show me how to heal myself*
- *Give me the courage to change my life*
- *Teach me how to love myself*
- *Help me understand my place in the world*
- *Help me surrender completely to the medicine*

Setting refers to where, when, and how you plan to have your journey. Some things to think about:

LOCATION: Use a safe, private, and comfy location. I have used my bed, sofa, and lounger on my deck. Have pillows and blankets nearby, and easy access to a toilet.

MUSIC: Create a playlist of favorite soothing/uplifting music. People recommend many types, including classical, Native American, ambient music/sounds, Georgian chants, New Age. Music really enhances these experiences. (See more here: https://happymag.tv/5-scientifically-approved-playlists-for-psychedelic-therapy/)

LIGHT: Some people use eye masks to block out stimuli, but I just close my eyes.

CLOTHING: Cozy clothing, with layers, works best as the medicine can affect your extremities.

TRIPSITTER: Especially for a first time, having a sober partner/friend/professional there to help you with the visions and journey can help alleviate challenging aspects of the experience.

MANAGING THE PSYCHEDELIC EXPERIENCE

If you are considering using a psychedelic medicine, it makes sense to do so using a trained facilitator in a secure and safe setting (such as in a psychedelic retreat or through a clinical trial) or in your home (or other safe location).

There's a lot of debate over the issue of a "bad trip," but one thing is certain: at higher dosages, psychedelics can push the limits of the mind as well as overload the emotions – resulting in a challenging trip, which is where a facilitator or tripsitter can help navigate potential difficulties and challenges.

At very low doses of these medicines, it may be safe to attempt a journey by yourself (but keep a friend and the number for the nonprofit Fireside Project – 623-473-7433 - on hand). However, at higher dosages, to do your best at harm reduction, it's a smart practice to have a sitter or facilitator or have the medicine administered to you at a healing center/clinic.

THE JOURNEY

Depending on the medicine and the dosage (and whether you decide to take a booster dose), the psychedelic journey can last from about half an hour to 12 hours. Please review the information on dosages and timing as you plan your work with these medicines.

Obviously, if you are at a retreat center, the facilitators should work with you on expectations about the medicine and the timing of your journey. Remember to

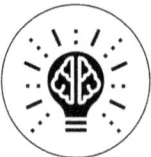

FUN FACT Besides psychedelics, here are a few other ways to improve neuroplasticity: exercise, meditation, and a healthier/nutrient-dense diet (especially avoiding sugar).

focus and meditate on your intention(s) as you head into the journey.

On a side note, expect to have some sort of purging experiences with these medicines – the process of eliminating energy, emotions, and trauma from the body – whether via traditional bodily experiences (vomiting and defecation, especially with Ayahuasca) or other purging, such as laughing, chanting, crying, shaking, sweating, yawning, and hacking.

As the journey winds down and comes to completion, you may feel exhausted, depleted, and ready to sleep/nap. In contrast, you may feel energized and alert and ready to make some changes. Regardless of how you feel, the next step – integration – is essential to the success of the medicine.

Finally, remember that you will be vulnerable for a few days after your journey, so plan to take it easy. Trust that the medicine worked and you just need time to process everything that happened. Most importantly, do NOT make any rash/major decisions during or immediately after your journey!

INSPIRING QUOTE "Psychedelics have been used by humans as tools for healing for millennia. Ample clinical trials have shown that these compounds are both safe and non-addictive if used correctly... I am convinced that psychedelic medicine will forever change our understanding of brain health."
– SONIA WEISS PICK

THE IMPORTANCE OF PSYCHEDELIC INTEGRATION: HOW & WHY

Consuming psychedelics without completing the integration of your journey into your regular life is like going to an expert for advice and then completely ignoring that advice.

One of the biggest misunderstandings of psychedelics is that they are a cure-all… that they are miracle medicines. Psychedelics are miraculous, but not magic pills. Psychedelics have proven power to change the brain and help people with numerous mental conditions, but their power comes from being a **tool** users can employ to heal themselves. **You are responsible for doing the work!**

Psychedelics open certain portals and increase awareness and knowledge of hidden and suppressed events/traumas – but participants MUST complete the work of integrating the psychedelic experiences into real change in their lives. Your goal should be making sense of the lessons and messages you received during your journey and determining how they can be applied to your everyday life.

Sometimes the lessons you are supposed to learn are brought out during the ceremony; others take reflection and time to come together into something meaningful. Regardless, psychedelic journeys provide you with an abundance of knowledge and insights, often an overwhelming amount.

Integration can be painful – intense/confusing realizations, acceptance, difficult/painful changes. Yet, integration is for the good – for leaving behind trauma and negative experiences and beginning anew.

Think of things this way: A psychedelic experience is the seed, your life the soil, integration like a blooming flower; as the petals open over time, the depth of your understanding, healing, and growth expands exponentially – so keep at it. To take this analogy one step deeper, as you are integrating your experience, you may need to change the "soil" in which you live – so that your flower blooms bigger, better, brighter.

The key thing to remember is integration is a process… which can take days, weeks, or months… and even years — depending on how much effort you put into it and how powerful the experiences. Integration involves reflecting, meditating, journaling, sharing, and action. Some parts of integration may be foreign to you – maybe even something you never expected. The critical part is to remember it is a process and to keep working at it. It may also take a bit of work to find what method works best for you; there's no rush, so the key is simply taking your time to sift through your journey and start processing and making connections. It took decades to construct what you are trying to unlearn; this process takes time; there is no shortcut to integrating.

Finally, remember that you must resist the temptation to push away the lessons and insights, to return to living your life as usual. As painful as some of these actions may be, as part of your integration, you may need to break old patterns/habits, break away from certain friends or family members – whatever it takes to foster the healing you need.

To truly experience complete integration, you should focus on three elements: first, dedicating time to mindfulness and gratitude for the life and people around you; second, physical/somatic integration that takes you to quiet places; and third, applying the lessons learned to your new life after psychedelics, typically through journaling.

FACILITATOR TIP Whether you are macrodosing or microdosing a psychedelic medicine, all experts agree that integrating your experience is essential to discovering more about yourself, your journey, your future direction.

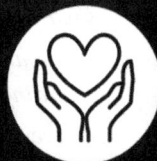

PERSONAL INTEGRATION TOOLS

This element of integration includes things like breathwork, yoga, massages, meditation, dance, time in nature (also called forest bathing).

The key is finding moments throughout your day to quietly reflect on your life, your journey, your future. Let ideas surface and simply make observations. Be in the moment as you participate in these activities.

> **INSPIRING QUOTE** "LSD shows you that there's another side to the coin, and you can't remember it when it wears off, but you know it. It reinforced my sense of what was important, creating great things instead of making money, putting things back into the stream of history and of human consciousness as much as I could." – STEVE JOBS

JOURNALING

In my mind, the best tool for integration is journaling. In fact, it's the best tool for your whole psychedelic experience, meaning once you decide to take a psychedelic medicine, you should begin journaling your thoughts, ideas, actions, etc.

You can journal in whatever way works for you – on an electronic device, in a book or binder, using words or a combination of words, and drawing/painting. The key is EXPRESSING all the details of what is going on in your head – from the journey and moving forward with your healing/transformation.

Once you have had some time to recover from the psychedelic journey, here are some journal questions/prompts that may help you with integration:

- *How do you feel overall?*
- *What was your overall impression of your journey?*
- *What things did you see and experience on your journey?*
- *What patterns were repeated throughout your journey?*
- *What are five words that best summarize your experience?*
- *What insights, visions, sensations did you experience?*
- *What feels like the most important things coming from your journey?*
- *What are you most grateful about regarding the experience?*
- *What parts of you did you let go of? Any parts of you that died?*
- *What part of the experience felt most challenging? What felt most rewarding?*
- *Are there any overarching themes to your experience?*
- *What are your most memorable moments, visions, insights?*

- *What feelings are most alive in your body as you reflect on your journey?*
- *What questions are still floating around your mind?*
- *Were your journey intentions met/answered?*
- *What attitudes and behaviors are no longer serving you?*
- *What am I holding onto – and what can I let go?*
- *What changes might you have to make in your life?*
- *What changes might you have to make in your digital life?*
- *What makes me happy – and what things do I want to avoid?*
- *Does my current work align with my newly discovered self? If not, what kind of work will fit?*
- *What kind of person are you now – and did you gain insights into changes you need to make?*
- *What kind of changes and conversations do you need to have with people after this experience?*
- *What kind of person do you want to be? What kind of relationships do you want? How will you make these ideas and changes a reality?*

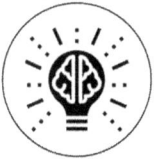

FUN FACT Integration comes from the Latin word integrare, which means forming or blending into a whole, or to complete. Psychedelic integration focuses on efforts to determine the wisdom from a psychedelic journey and bring it fully into our waking lives. It's about changing perspectives and creating a path to change.

DON'T IGNORE OR PUT OFF JOURNALING! We have a friend who went on his first medicinal psychedelic journey with psilocybin in which he spent the entire journey maniacally laughing and apologizing to his spouse about his poor English and grammar. When we asked him about the meaning of these actions and whether he had journaled about them, he look perplexed, replying, "Why would I journal when nothing happened?" He didn't realize everything that happens during a journey has meaning and should be documented and reviewed.

You'll also want to integrate spiritually and emotionally.

With higher doses of medicine, people often experience spiritual encounters, and it's important to journal about them and their meaning. These encounters may change our beliefs in God, about spirituality, about universal connectedness and consciousness.

With higher doses of the medicine, people have deeply emotional journeys – with results ranging from grief, joy, gratitude, forgiveness – and it is equally important to process these emotional outcomes.

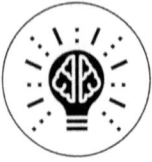

FUN FACT Researchers are studying the use of MDMA-assisted therapy for autistic adults who have moderate to severe social anxiety. One study showed that MDMA causes one to more accurately deduce social and emotional information and its mental states, which can be of great benefit to autistic people. (https://embrace-autism.com/mdma-assisted-therapy-for-autistic-people/)

COMMUNITY

One final note about integration. You should not – and some would say cannot – do it alone.

Whether it's the people who also participated in the psychedelic journey or your significant other or a community of others who have had psychedelic experiences, you need to seek out community… seek out others to share stories and struggles. You could also consider hiring an integration coach if connecting with a like-minded community is not an option.

One excellent online community for meeting others who have had psychedelic journeys is Empathic Health (https://www.empathic.health/), whose mission is to "craft the best healing community in the world for our members, and to have fun doing it."

Another great resource for discovering like-minded people near you is by finding and joining one or more psychedelic societies. (Find one list here: https://www.pendulum.org/psychedelic-societies/)

HOW TO HAVE A MEDICINAL PSYCHEDELIC JOURNEY

As the legal landscape continues to evolve, some of these methods will change as well. For now, here are the ways in which one can seek healing and transformation through psychedelics:

- *Join a clinical trial (https://psychedelic.support/resources/how-to-join-psychedelic-clinical-trial/)*
- *Go abroad to one of many retreats, including Europe, Mexico, and South America (https://retreat.guru/)*
- *Attend an underground healing center ceremony (but only after carefully vetting)*
- *Find a qualified psychedelic-assisted therapist*
- *Hire a professional guide or tripsitter*
- *Source the medicine from the underground marketplace*

EXPERT GUEST FINAL WORDS ON MACRODOSING

AN ACCIDENTAL PSYCHONAUT... LEADS TO LASTING TRANSFORMATION

By Matt Zemon, MSc

I am an accidental psychonaut. I was never much of a drug user, except for a few experiences with cannabis when I was younger. In 2019, I had the opportunity to experience a guided psilocybin (magic mushroom) journey, and it completely changed my worldview. Almost 30 years after my last science class, I went back to school for a Master's degree in Psychology and Neuroscience of Mental Health and have committed myself to better understanding the biological and psychological foundation upon which psychedelic psychotherapy is building.

It was a difficult road that led me to my first macrodose experience with psychedelic medicine, but not an uncommon one. Like many others, it stemmed from grief and trauma. When I was 22 my mom died. She was just 49 years old. When she passed, it felt like a piece of my heart was ripped from my chest. I felt empty. I lost any faith I had in God. But over time, life moved on. I began a career, got married, had kids; all while missing my mom.

And it's easy to box up those feelings and put them in a dark place somewhere where you can ignore them and pretend they don't exist. Until you can't anymore.

In 2019, some good friends of mine suggested that I try a guided psychedelic experience with a macrodose of psilocybin. I didn't even know what psilocybin was or why I'd want to try it. But my friends talked about how much they – and others – had learned from these experiences. They described it as going on a trip in your mind. I liked learning. I liked traveling. I figured, "why not?"

Going into the experience, I didn't really know what to expect, but our guide told us that we would be safe. He told us that we may have a challenging experience and that if that happened, to try and open ourselves up to whatever was causing fear or anxiety and what we were meant to learn from those feelings. We ate the mushrooms and practiced some meditation.

INSPIRING QUOTE "Some people have referred to iboga as the 'Mt. Everest' of psychedelic medicines. Iboga can be a rigorous physical, mental, and spiritual journey – and yet there is always a profound and loving intelligence at play, even through highly challenging moments. Iboga may perhaps be the most psychologically complex and confrontational of all medicines, inviting us to examine and release beliefs, coping mechanisms, personality structures, or habits that no longer serve us – or that are not rooted in truth. We may find ourselves with a new world view." – ELIZABETH BAST, BWITI IBOGA PROVIDER

75

What I experienced next is hard to put into words. I was gone. It was as if I had melted into the ground and was watching and feeling the world breathe. I became aware of my grandparents and great-grandparents and all of the people I was connected to in the world. I felt unconditional love like I never remember feeling before. And I felt safe – truly safe. It brought me to the realization that I hadn't ever been able to truly share love, even with my wife and children. I was living my life scared. Scared of really living, scared of dying.

And then, I saw my mom. And felt her presence. Instantly I understood that she wasn't gone; she'd be part of me forever. I could pull a string from her to me, and then to my children. We were all connected. For the first time in the 24 years since my mom passed, my heart felt full again. I understood deeply in my soul that we are all connected, and we are all part of something bigger. I remembered true joy, and I was no longer afraid of dying, living, or loving.

Over the years since my first macrodose experience, I've immersed myself in the world of psychedelic medicine and studied the transformative and healing potential of entheogenic substances, particularly the research around the practice of macrodosing with psychedelic substances as a means to achieve positive and lasting spiritual change and healing.

My research has led me to publish my first book on psychedelic medicine, *Psychedelics for Everyone: A Beginner's Guide to these Powerful Medicines for Anxiety, Depression, Addiction, PTSD, and Expanding Consciousness.* I don't believe everyone should take psychedelics, but I do believe that psychedelics are for everyone. There is a lot of information on psychedelics available, but much of it is not written for the average person. My book is an attempt to gather accurate information on a number of different psychedelic medicines and put it into one place for easy reference that the average person can understand.

For my first macrodose experience, I took just over 5 grams of dried mushrooms. Regarding what the correct dose for a macrodose is, Johns Hopkins University has conducted extensive research on the appropriate dosage to offer users the positive benefits of psilocybin while minimizing the negative effects that can come from a "bad trip" (Griffiths et al., 2011). What they found in 2011 is that at very high doses (30 mg/70 kg, p.o., meaning "per oral" or by mouth),

FACILITATOR TIP If possible, schedule your journey for a time when you can take several days off work (and life) to rest, relax, unwind, recuperate – without having the stress of work or the need to face people.

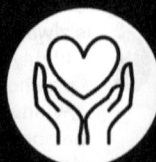

volunteers reported spiritually significant happenings, but almost a third of participants also reported suffering from anxiety, stress, and fear episodes during the experience. The second highest dose (20 mg/70 kg, p.o.), however, resulted in all the positive benefits, with none of the negative effects. According to the lead author of the study, this moderately high dose, sometimes called a hero dose, provides a "high probability of a profound and beneficial experience, a low enough probability of psychological struggle, and very little risk of any actual harm."

In 2021, the researchers studied weight-adjusted vs. fixed-dosing approaches and concluded that the convenience of fixed-dose administration outweighs any potential advantage of weight-adjusting dosage (Garcia-Romeu, Barrett, Carbonaro, Johnson, & Griffiths, 2021). Across a wide range of body weights ranging from 100 pounds to 250 pounds, the optimal dose was 25 mg, equating to 4.5 grams of dried Psilocybe Cubensis, the most common type of psilocybin mushroom. (Psilocybe Cubensis contains approximately .56% psilocybin when dried.)

There are currently more than 300 centers for psychedelic studies and psychedelic research at major academic institutions across the world, and there are many philosophies regarding who should have access to psychedelics and competing interests as to how. While the future of psychedelic medicine in America is still to be determined, the results from the research happening are groundbreaking, and politicians and voters on both sides of the aisle are supportive.

I grew up in the "just say no" 1970s and 1980, and when I started my journey, I had no idea about the potential for transformative healing that can come from psychedelic medicine.

One macrodose changed the way I see the world. While my interest in psychedelic medicine started by accident, I share this story in the hopes that it will open minds to the possibilities of psychedelic medicine so that others can enter with intentionality.

REFERENCES:

Garcia-Romeu, A., Barrett, F. S., Carbonaro, T. M., Johnson, M. W., & Griffiths, R. R. (2021). Optimal dosing for psilocybin pharmacotherapy: Considering weight-adjusted and fixed dosing approaches. *Journal of psychopharmacology (Oxford, England), 35*(4), 353-361. doi:10.1177/0269881121991822

Griffiths, R. R., Johnson, M. W., Richards, W. A., Richards, B. D., McCann, U., & Jesse, R. (2011). Psilocybin occasioned mystical-type experiences: immediate and persisting dose-related effects. *Psychopharmacology (Berl), 218*(4), 649-665. doi:10.1007/s00213-011-2358-5

PART TWO:

REAL STORIES OF HEALING AND TRANSFORMATIONAL JOURNEYS

THE STORIES

This section of the book is the heart of why you and I are here. These stories are raw and direct – and share as many details as possible so that you get a true sense of what it's like taking these medicines.

You will find stories by people from all walks of life and all ages… and while the psychedelic industry has been more white-male-oriented, you'll find stories from all genders and races/ethnicities. The stories come from people who were seeking healing, people who were seeking transformation, and people seeking the Divine.

You are invited to take a deep dive into the healing stories of these courageous people.

CHAPTER FOUR

Healing Story #1
Just Say YES! Psychedelics Saved
My Life – and My Family

STORYTELLER: Allison, Female, White/Caucasian, Gen X, military spouse

MEDICINE CONSUMED: 1ˢᵗ day was Pharmaceutical Grade MDMA and psilocybin; 2ⁿᵈ day was 5-MeO-DMT

DOSAGE: Total 4.5 grams psilocybin (1ˢᵗ dose 3.5 grams and 2ⁿᵈ dose 1 gram a few hours later) and 185 mg of MDMA (1ˢᵗ dose 125 mg and 2ⁿᵈ dose 60mg a few hours later)

FOCUS/GOAL/INTENTION: I was so desperate at this time, that I needed to go to live, I needed to do this to make it to another day and I had no idea why I was stuck where I was. I had no love and no life left. I was a shell of a person and this was my last HOPE.

BEST PART OF THIS JOURNEY: After breaking through and letting my guard down, I was able to see, feel, touch, hear, and experience so much LOVE.

BIGGEST CHALLENGE OF JOURNEY: Getting there, I almost didn't make it. I almost didn't even let go once I took the medicine.

....

PROFOUND HEALING JOURNEY STORY DETAILS

Have you ever just said YES? It's pretty invigorating and so powerful. Before this trip, I said NO a lot. I said NO because I was scared. I said NO because I thought I was not good enough and didn't need it. I said NO because I didn't like too much change. I said NO because I didn't love myself enough.

My psychedelic journey began in a facility in Costa Rica in which I was fortunate to be paired with a Gold Star wife (who had lost her husband), a veteran, and me, a SEAL wife – the first women's retreat for the center. (The three of us had never met each other before this experience, but we are soul sisters and have a deep connection after our journeys. We were meant to be on this healing journey together.) The center included coaches, doctors, and nurses who would watch over our care.

I was scared shitless. My ego was so large – and mind you I had to taper off all my prescription medications before arriving at the center… so I wasn't in a good spot at all.

I had so many questions to ask the medicine. SO many. I had so many expectations. You should never go in with expectations and that is what everyone told me, but it was hard. It was really hard. I wrote down intentions and questions and I truly got them all answered in one word…. **LOVE**! That's all that matters.

The day I took the medicine, I remember thinking, what the hell am I doing? I mean, I have five beautiful children at home and here I am in the middle of the jungle, where I don't know anyone and am about to take drugs.

What am I doing? But I had gotten to a point where there was nowhere left to go. So I had to just take a leap of faith. What else do I have to lose?

The first day started with us sitting in the circle saying prayers and being smudged (to clear away negative energy). We didn't have to say a word. We were holding space for each other. We were there. We all said YES. We all wanted to be there to start a journey, a journey we would have never imagined.

I knew that once I took these medicines, there was no going back. My babies and husband were in the U.S. and I was there in the jungle and there was no going back. Just say YES, just say YES….is all I kept saying! These girls taught me that! My family is a wonderful and powerful group and truly woven together like branches on a tree.

On that first day, I was given 3.5 grams of psilocybin containing mushrooms and 125 mg of pharmaceutical grade MDMA. Two hours later I opted to take a supplemental dose of each medicine (1 gram of mushrooms and 60 mg of MDMA). This is a healing treatment using entheogens that lasts about 6-8 hours. That first day, with the MDMA, which is a heart-opener, was so powerful – and it is NOT the ecstasy you go out and take at raves.

After the medicine was ingested, we were brought back to three mattresses laid closely together with beautiful flower arrangements at the top of each. Eye masks were laid out and then the most beautiful music was playing in the background. It was so peaceful. I was still so anxious.

I felt nothing. Was this working? Was I immune to this medicine because of all of the benzos I took for years or the drugs I put into my body in a non-therapeutic way? Would this work and what is going to happen?

I can remember lying down with eye shades and music, just lying there and hearing the birds, sounds of nature; it was beautiful. I can also remember crossing my legs and thinking, "This isn't working; it isn't working." The control freak in me and my ego... I kept saying to myself, surrender, surrender. Let the medicine do its job.

With my right hand I started clenching my stomach and crying. Why? Why all the tears? Why am I holding my stomach? Am I scared for my babies? Do I need to be a better mom? Am I not present enough? Why? All of these questions are still in my head. I haven't surrendered yet. I am still aware. I am still here and I have not gone deeper.

Then it hit me. I heard her. I heard a little girl... and this voice, it kept saying "Mommy, mommy." And I wondered what was going on. Was it one of my kids trying to talk to me? But she kept at it, saying "Mommy, mommy, I am ok."

I surrendered to her... to HOPE, but I was still clenching my stomach; it almost hurt. What is happening to me? Hope began to say to me, "Mommy, come with me. Mommy, I'm OK – and I want you to see, I want you to see the beauty mommy."

I sat up and immediately wrote "HOPE" on my arm... and she was the little girl from when I had an abortion at 17. And she came to me in the journey and kept repeating, "I'm OK. You can let go now." She had opened this door of love – and surrender.

I had not thought of about that abortion for years and years and years. It was shoved so far down inside that as soon as that door opened, she took me on the entire journey of my life... and coming out of that journey, I knew that I had to love myself... that was the entire journey. I had to love myself.

I did not love myself because of what happened when I was younger and it just kept piling up and piling up... and I never

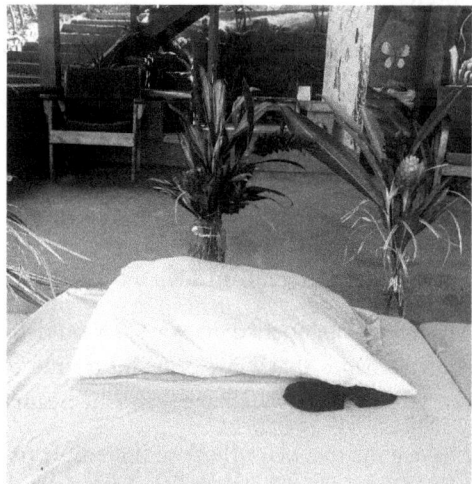

A photo of Allison's ceremonial space.

let anyone – not my husband nor my children – love me. I had a wall up the entire time.

That journey saved my life. It saved my children's lives. It saved my marriage. During this journey, I found LOVE. I found love for myself and for my husband. I saw my husband's love for me. I never saw my husband in my visions, but I saw his love. Does that make sense? It was just there and with the forgiveness I had for myself and my abortion, knowing Hope was OK and feeling that love, I went through this magical place.

I had so much joy and love running through my veins, I never wanted it to end. It was breathtaking. I was in heaven and all because I said YES.

KEY INSIGHT: But, remember, the medicine is just a tool. It's a tool to fast track where you need to be, but these tools... you don't come home and you're changed and you're integrating into this beautiful place – because the world does not change... the world's still a shitshow at times. We need to integrate these fully experiences.

I feel like the world should have to integrate to us. That the world needs to take psychedelics and then the world would integrate to us – and we would not need to integrate to the world.

Why? Because there is so much more work that needs to be done. Since this healing experience, I have done a few smaller journeys – to help me when I get stuck in a spot.

This experience allowed me to love myself so that I could react to things differently... so that I could see love differently... so that I could accept love differently.

On that journey, I was also told I should start the Hope Project. I have made it my purpose, my passion, to connect other spouses, other female veterans, and Gold Star wives to psychedelics, but also to be there for them with prep and integration coaching.

I left Costa Rica a different woman. I mean, if you met me the week before this experience and then met me afterward.... you would think I was the same, but I'm not. I'm different. In such a beautiful way I am different.

My heart was opened in ways I would have never imagined. My mind was shown images that have been inside me for years. I have seen heaven. I love everything so much. I have seen true beauty.

I have gone to a place that's so incredibly magical... And all of this because I said YES. I was brave, I was strong, I conquered my fears and I said YES... and you can too!

PERSONAL BACKGROUND

Everything about this journey starts when my husband decided he wanted to become a Navy SEAL. I supported his decision, but did not know how hard it would be to be married to a SEAL.

Once he became a SEAL, people would tell me I was so lucky to be married to a "hero."

Yet the reality was he was gone for about 300 days a year. We moved quite often, now in our 20th home. We also had five children during this time… and I just have to say it's hard on the family.

The SEAL members get a lot of support, but the wives do not. Oh, we wives would have a dinner now and again, but they often turned so negative, that I just did not want to go anymore… so I began feeling quite alone.

When my husband would go to his next deployment, I would definitely numb myself with alcohol. I was also on benzos [Benzodiazepines, often prescribed for anxiety] for 16 years. I then started abusing the benzos so that I could just make it through to the next day.

I stopped watching the news. I started wondering if/when I was going to get that knock on the door – telling me that my husband is not coming home. But then I started thinking, maybe I do want that knock on the door because I don't want to live like this anymore… and then how awful I felt for feeling that way – like I actually want this to end because maybe then I could move on with my life.

The command used to tell us that we have to hold it together at home – because if we are not together, then the guys are going to be affected and be bad operators. And frankly? That sucked. Trying to be a mom to five children and hold it together and shove everything down.

And when I went into the marriage, forget about all the traumas I had – that everyone has – and forget about the traumas that happened to me as a child or later as a teenager. That trauma had to be shoved so deep down inside so that I could hold it together on the outside.

And how did I hold it together? By taking a combination of benzos, antidepressants, and alcohol – and that was for 16 years.

When my husband retired, I was so excited because I thought it was finally my time. My turn to hold down a job. My turn to find friends. To maybe be able to go back to school. To be in a home and have it feel like an actual home.

The reality was it was not like that at all. It was me picking up the pieces – because my husband did not have his purpose or his passion.

I admit that I was not a good wife. It was a volatile relationship still running on medication and alcohol.

He then got to go on a healing journey with Ibogaine in Mexico – and came back changed – but I was not this ball of love to come back to. I was mad, angry, resentful. Why did he get to feel this way while I was struggling – what about me? And then I began to feel more awful for feeling that way.

In some ways, nothing had changed – and I wondered when I was ever going to get off this hamster wheel.

I wanted NOTHING to do with psychedelics. I thought, "This is bullshit." I just need to take my medication. I went to my psychologist and the answer was to increase my dosage.

I remember the day when everything changed like it was yesterday. It was on a small farm we had in Connecticut. I was sitting in our horse's stall and just broke down and called him and said to him, "If you do not get me on a plane or to a doctor soon, I am not sure I can make it to tomorrow."

I had thoughts, constant thoughts, of killing myself… in many, many different ways. But I also had five beautiful children and a husband… and this beautiful home in Connecticut… we had everything.

So, kicking and screaming my husband got me on a plane to Costa Rica. I almost did not get on the second plane… but so thankful I did!

EDITOR'S NOTES:

KEY TAKEAWAYS FROM ALLISON'S STORY

- Turning away from the fears and misinformation related to psychedelics – and embracing the medicine and potential healing – can result in complete transformations.
- We all have hidden (or forgotten) trauma from earlier in our lives – and the power of these psychedelic medicines is that they shred those walls and barriers and expose the trauma, allowing one to finally face the issue – and move forward.
- While every psychedelic experience is unique, the journeys often end with a sense of hope, love, connectedness to the world/universe.
- People who are self-medicating (whether prescribed or not) with benzos and antidepressants, as well as with alcohol and other drugs, need to slowly reduce that consumption prior to taking a psychedelic journey – weaning off those bad drugs is essential to the success of the psychedelic medicines.

OTHER DETAILS

Allison Wilson is Founder & President of The Hope Project. She currently lives on a small farm outside of Denver where she gets to unwind, relax, and enjoy many animals including dogs, cats, horses, chickens, ducks and goats! Hope Project: https:// thehope-project.org/

CHAPTER FIVE

Healing Story #2
A Combat Veteran's Journey Home -
Reconnecting Heart and Mind

STORYTELLER: Ryan, Male, White/Caucasian, Millennial, U.S. Marine

MEDICINE CONSUMED: Ibogaine and 5-MeO-DMT

DOSAGE: 800 mg Ibogaine; unsure of 5-MeO-DMT

FOCUS/GOAL/INTENTION: To reconnect with myself and the world around me. I also wanted the trauma to end with me… not passed to my kids.

BEST PART OF THIS JOURNEY: Reconnecting with my higher self (my true self) and my life's purpose

BIGGEST CHALLENGE OF JOURNEY: Ibogaine is physically grueling. The experience for me was >12 hours

....

PROFOUND HEALING JOURNEY STORY DETAILS

How do you even begin to share an experience that can only be described as ineffable? Words have the ability to be extremely powerful, but they're merely symbols used to convey complex emotions and thoughts. Words are linear tools for a multidimensional reality. They will always fall short of the desired impact. Nevertheless, I will give it my best shot.

In November 2021, I met up with Michael "Punky" Higgs, retired Navy SEAL and Director of Operations for Mission Within, and the other service members as we headed for a retreat house in Mexico. We all were welcomed with loving, open arms.

For those unfamiliar with Ibogaine, it's a plant medicine that does come with some medical risks. However, Mission Within has a comprehensive intake process that medically screens applicants for risks – such as prescription contraindications and/or existing medical issues.

To say that the experience with Ibogaine was challenging would be a gross understatement. There is a higher intelligence contained within the plant that gives you exactly what you need – not what you want or think you need. While everyone's experiences are a bit different, for me, there were almost no visual or auditory hallucinations.

The medicine came on hard and strong. I felt it start at the tips of my toes and work its way through my entire body as if it was performing a scan to identify troubled areas. I knew exactly what areas of my body it was working on, but my physical body was in some sort of paralysis.

As the medicine worked in my body, I began to ask the Ibogaine specific questions and it would answer me with clarity that could only be interpreted energetically. Not with the usual five senses. I can only describe it as a sense of **_knowing_**. This part of the journey lasted about 4 to 6 hours.

For me, the experience was physically challenging, but the medicine was also kind and gentle. However, I achieved a sense of surrender that I didn't even know was possible. Right when my ego said, "OK, OK, I surrender. I can't take anymore" I moved directly into the next phase of the journey.

This next phase, lasting about 6 hours, I can only describe as deep, quiet, and contemplative. The medicine was still working on my body, but my mind was still. During this time, I constructed the life I wanted, the person I wanted to be, and what tangible steps I needed to take to arrive there.

My ego had been beaten into submission and I could only watch as a bystander as I slowly transcended it. I cried and cried. Then the cries turned to laughter. The laughter turned to the most powerful energy… it was Love. I felt like light was beaming from my body. Then, as quickly as it came in, the Ibogaine subsided.

The next 10 to 12 hours were physically and emotionally challenging. I couldn't eat, couldn't drink, and I could barely muster the energy to get to the bathroom. Never in my life (that I can recall) had I been free of my ego. This period was quiet contemplation; all was quiet – no thoughts, just feelings.

After doing some recovery and integration from the Ibogaine experience, we had a 5-MeO-DMT – the God Molecule – ceremony on Day 3. This medicine shattered every paradigm… every construct … every framework into a billion pieces.

We started with a small "handshake" dose to help familiarize our bodies with the medicine. Then it was my turn for a full dose. The medicine woman told me to count backward from 10 once I had inhaled the medicine, but before I got anywhere with the countdown, my world started vibrating, and immediately after exhaling, I was launched like a rocket into a place that doesn't exist on our usual plane of consciousness. I hate to even call it a place because it was everywhere and nowhere at the same time.

It sounds crazy, but my physical form simply disintegrated. My body was lying on the bed, but my soul – my energetic self was in the most beautiful place. I was with God… with Christ consciousness. Nothing existed in this space but unconditional love. *I felt immersed in an ocean of bliss.* The concept of "Ryan" no longer existed and I didn't feel attached to it. I don't remember feeling any discomfort or fear… just love… love… love. Then I began to return back from the medicine.

I signaled for, and received, an even larger dose. This time when the medicine woman finished counting down, everything ceased to exist. I was back in space, this time merging into Oneness with God. I looked around as my energy exploded into billions of particles over and over again. Then God reached his hand into my energy fields and began to remove all the blockages.

Every last shred of guilt, shame, hate, rage, and fear was stripped from my energetic being and discarded into the ether. In the presence of unconditional love, they held no power and merged into love.

I felt as if God had spoken to me. It wasn't auditory, but I knew there was a message. The downloads came hard and fast. Then I felt as if my body was hooked to an electric grid and pumped full of eternal and unconditional love. Afterward, I found myself lying there on the bed in a puddle of joyful tears.

I felt as if the weight of the world had been lifted from my chest. I breathed in deeply and took the fullest breath possible. Every fear-based emotion had been lifted and replaced with pure love and gratitude.

PERSONAL BACKGROUND

I was raised just outside New York City, so my story has to start with 9/11. I enlisted with the U.S. Marine Corps Infantry, First Battalion Second Marines, with which I served multiple deployments to Iraq – and witnessed so much carnage, of my fellow Marines as well as countless civilians. Little did I know it then, but that trauma became a cancer that almost ruined me. I learned much later, I was suffering from "moral injury." I became a shell of a human being.

Because of my years of service, for the better part of the last 18 years, I struggled with PTSD, depression, anxiety, and a plethora of issues resulting from multiple traumatic brain injuries. I had constant panic attacks that led to hospital visits. I had trouble sleeping. I felt alone in the world. I self-medicated with alcohol. I had serious, daily suicidal ideations. I developed a hatred for myself. At times, I felt like a sociopath conjuring lies to serve as "emotions" because I couldn't connect with anyone or anything… most importantly my Higher Self.

Superficially, I "appeared" well put together but, on the inside, I had burnt down to a few remaining embers of *Truth*. Those embers were on the brink of being suffocated by shame, anger, hate, sadness, and loneliness when my world imploded and I fell flat on my face. I hit rock bottom. On the brink of losing EVERYTHING, a voice inside me quietly said, "You are a person worth saving."

I spent the next 3 years listening to that voice and began piecing my life back together. Not as it was, but as I wanted it to be. I had to embark on a hero's journey to reconnect my heart and mind. I had neglected myself for so long that it was a real struggle. How could I provide love to a person that I held nothing but contempt for? Well, I started small. I began meditating twice a day. That led to breathwork. That led to float tank therapy, somatic therapy, and gratitude practices. I even was invited to participate in a Lakota sweat lodge ceremony. I began to feel OK sitting with myself.

I wish I could tell you that all of those practices were enough to get me where I am today – but I still had baggage to shed, social and spiritual conditioning to undo, and armor to remove. I was aware of the negative loops playing, but regardless of the efforts I put into rewriting them, I still felt lost and alone.

After much reflection and discussion with mentors, I became aware that my body was holding on to deep-seated trauma that had to be released.

I'm a highly analytical person who structures his world through the application of frameworks and proven models. So… I began to research plant medicines. I read book after book. Listened to podcast after podcast. My paradigm was quickly shifting because I rediscovered the *Truths* that were always within me. I became a sponge and soaked up as much healing as I possibly could, but there was still this cloud of pain and sorrow following me around. As they say, what you resist, persists.

Amazingly, I had several opportunities to sit with various plant medicines, but I just didn't feel called to them. I had heard over and over from the plant medicine community that if I didn't feel called to the medicine, not to partake. The right plant medicine will find me when I am truly ready and open to the experience… happily, a close friend and mentor, Dr. Martin Polanco, founder of *The Mission Within*, reached out to me, which led me to my healing journeys.

Today, after completing all the preliminary work and then receiving the healing from the Ibogaine and 5-MeO-DMT, I am still integrating the experience…

and that integration will last a lifetime. My life is unrecognizable. I'm simply not the person I was. I've become the best version of myself possible.

FINAL THOUGHTS: To all the amazing veteran organizations sponsoring plant medicine opportunities, thank you! The countless hours you dedicate to raising awareness, philanthropy, and dollars for clinical research are not going unnoticed. You are saving lives!

These medicines are powerful catalysts for healing – but they are not light switches – we still have to do the work to truly heal ourselves.

Just know that these medicines – in the right set and setting, with the right people and right support, with a clear intention, we can manifest a beautiful life for ourselves. We are the medicine that we are searching for.

EDITOR'S NOTES:

KEY TAKEAWAYS FROM RYAN'S STORY

- Don't go chasing these medicines. Time and time again, it has been shown anecdotally that the medicine will find you when you are ready to accept it.
- Finding the correct medicine(s) and the correct facility are essential to helping you achieve successful healing.
- Never give up on healing – and finding a healing modality for you. These medicines are powerful tools, but the real healing comes from the person willing to put in the work to get that end result.
- Veterans have several options for healing through plant medicines and psychedelics, including: The Mission Within, Heroic Hearts Project, Veterans Exploring Treatment Solutions (VETS), Veterans of War, The Hope Project, Beckley Retreats, and SABE.

OTHER DETAILS

Ryan Roberts, MBA, after more than a decade of military and healthcare leadership, is currently an operations consultant with The Mission Within. Mission Within: https://missionwithin.org/

The song that came on when I returned was In Dreams, *by Jai-Jagdeesh. It truly tied a bow on the entire weekend for me. It was a synthesis of every download…*

Know you are loved…
Rest in peace
Dream your sweet dreams
'Til your soil is released
Beloved child
My heart is yours
Beloved child
My heart is yours
Beloved child
Go out and open doors
With your love
With your faith
With your compassion
With your grace
Oh, with your grace…
Beloved child
You are the light of the world
Beloved child…
Go out, spread light to the world
Be strong, be kind, be brave
Know your mind
Know that you're divine
Know that it's alright to be afraid.

CHAPTER SIX

Healing Story #3
Desperation Turns to Healing and Relief

STORYTELLER: Crystal, Female, White/Caucasian, Gen X

MEDICINE Consumed: Psilocybin (dried, ground, soaked in lemon juice and then steeped into a mint tea)

DOSAGE: 3 grams

FOCUS/GOAL/INTENTION: I was just desperate to feel better overall. Actually, without intention, this first experience was the one that precipitated my road to sobriety (from alcohol).

BEST PART OF THIS JOURNEY: This experience was like 15 years of therapy in one fell swoop. I immediately felt lighter, happier, and more at ease than I had in as long as I can remember. I felt hopeful.

BIGGEST CHALLENGE OF JOURNEY: I was terrified going into it. I nearly had a panic attack right out of the gate but I had ingested the tea and there was no going back so I just calmed myself down and went on the journey.

....

PROFOUND HEALING JOURNEY STORY DETAILS

A few weeks prior to my journey, I had a DUI. It was my second one (in a decade plus) and I was DISGUSTED with myself. I was already struggling mentally (depression, which was part of the reason that I was self-medicating with alcohol) but after the DUI I was struggling with suicidal ideation.

I knew that I needed to take it seriously because I had survived a suicide attempt 13 years prior. Therapy was not helping me and I was desperate for ANYTHING that would work to help me feel better so that I could stop thinking about dying all day, every day.

I found two playlists on Spotify that were recommended (one was based on playlists used by Imperial College of London, the other was based on a Johns Hopkins playlist). I already had a face mask that I sleep with every night so I was comfortable with wearing that. I made sure that I had fully charged earbuds and that I had an extra set of wired earbuds, just in case. I made sure that my room was cozy and that I had everything I thought I would need. I prepared and ingested the tea, put on a face mask, and started the journey.

I immediately started to panic after I consumed the medicine and I was deeply concerned with how this panic would affect my journey. I remembered something I had read/saw that suggested that when faced with negative feelings (like panic) you should ask yourself why you are feeling this way and then address it. It's a really simple way to explain a slightly deeper process but it worked. I was just scared of the unknown so I told myself that everything would be okay, I was safe, and everything was going to be okay if I trusted myself... so I did.

I feel like the playlist was extremely integral to my experience and that it was the perfect playlist for my first time (I used the Spotify playlist titled, "Psilocybin-assisted Therapy, v.2.4 by Ugis Salna). Once things were underway, I started feeling at ease. I took my mask off and the first thing that I saw was my ceiling fan, which seemed to be reaching out for me... and that made me giggle. My cat was lying next to me and when I looked at him, I didn't really like his face (I LOVE him but he has markings that made him look like a skull) but I loved the feel of his fur and he started purring when I touched him so I felt cozy from that.

One thing that stood out to me as odd (in the moment) was that instead of seeing colors/fractals as everyone describes, I felt like I was standing on a balcony with the breeze blowing long, flowing curtains all around me (a fan next to my bed was running) and in front of me were all beautiful scenes from nature that I had seen throughout the years. (We take a week-long trip every year where I ride on the back of a motorcycle and I was seeing what reminded me of images from those trips and time that we had spent at the beach – no people, just scenery.)

As things progressed, I needed to go to the restroom and I started getting scared again... scared to walk, scared to see myself in a mirror (which I had been told could be terrifying) and scared to take my mask off. In that moment, almost as if it was meant to happen, the playlist changed to a drum beat and I felt "guided" to the bathroom. I discovered that I loved the pattern on my toilet paper and found a new appreciation for water when washing my hands.

I felt safe after that experience so I went down to my kitchen to get water. (I use a Soda Stream to carbonate my water which was a whole NEW, fantastic, experience...I love bubbles!) After getting water, I went back upstairs to climb back into the nest I had made for myself in bed... and this is where things became intense.

After putting my mask back on and settling in, I was no longer alone in nature, I was standing in a memory.

My stepsister was murdered many years back and I guess I needed to address it because suddenly I was standing in our old yard with her and we were "talking." I could feel the breeze, see things that I had long forgotten about: a corn decoration hanging in our screened porch of all things, a kiddy pool we had been playing in, our Barbies, etc., I remember subconsciously communicating to her about how sad I felt for what happened to her and how terrible it was for her family. We were not that close as adults but we had been closer as children and I addressed that with her.

After some time, I remembered having a really good cry "with" her and then it was over. I felt calm and at ease.

After more time passed, I was feeling a bit braver and compelled to go find some photographs (I'm not sure why, I was just led to it... for lack of a better description). I gathered what I wanted (and a couple of other things I had found along the way) and went back to bed where I started looking at everything.

One of the things I found was a paper my son had written (with the help of a teacher) about what I meant to him... and I lost it and started sobbing. After that, I felt like this (looking at things) may be a bit much for me, so I put everything aside, put my mask back on, and went back to just focusing on the playlist.

Not much later, I felt that I was "coming out" of the journey and starting to feel more "normal." I'd say maybe 40 minutes later, I was out totally done with the trip and went to sit on my deck. I started smoking a joint and contemplating everything that had just occurred... and smiling – which was something that I had not done genuinely in quite some time.

The next morning, I felt really alive. I was grateful for the experience and eager to discuss it with my partner who was heading back from a camping trip. I was unsure how he would feel about it but I felt empowered enough to say that this was something that I WAS going to continue. His response was that if it made me feel this good, I should definitely do it.

PERSONAL BACKGROUND

My mom had me when she was 16 years old, by one day. She met my birth father when he was in the Marines (Camp LeJeune) and moved here to Kansas City to raise me.

My father was an alcoholic and was abusive to her. (I am fairly sure that he had an undiagnosed mental illness.) He eventually left her for another woman (with kids our age). My mom worked multiple jobs to keep us fed and in our house.

I didn't realize it until I was older, but I was very stressed as a child. I pulled out my hair (on my head, my eyelashes, and eyebrows) and I was always careful to do everything just right.

Because of all of these things, I carry a lot of trauma from my childhood that psilocybin has helped me address.

And, sadly, because psilocybin is illegal in Missouri, I have not found a reliable, regular source of mushrooms so I cannot microdose them like I would like to try, so I stick to quarterly consumption. Not every journey has been as enlightening as my first but there is always something valuable that occurs.

SIDE NOTE: I love documentaries, especially about nature/medicine, and had come across a documentary (*A New Understanding: The Science of Psilocybin*) that struck a nerve with me so I started seeking any information on psilocybin that I could find and I lost myself in it. I was just starting as a professional in the cannabis industry and was already feeling PISSED about all of the misinformation I was told in school about cannabis and now I was feeling the same way about psychedelics. If I am honest, I kind of felt like what do I have to lose by trying psilocybin? So, I did!

If you are interested in trying psilocybin, please do not hesitate. Do your research, find someone who can sit with you, but DO IT! I am so frustrated and angry about the lies I was told about psychedelics and I want to share how beneficial they are with anyone willing to listen.

I went from literally wanting to die, every single day, to thriving and I know that psilocybin played a tremendous role in getting me here.

FINAL THOUGHTS: I've really struggled with mental health because I was already told that I wasn't "strong enough." After I attempted suicide, I refused to let my parents come to visit me in the hospital until I was told that I couldn't leave until they did. After my attempt, I went to nursing school at a Catholic college – and I went to mass every day… and I needed that at the time. I've since become less religious but I am spiritual.

EDITOR'S NOTES:

KEY TAKEAWAYS FROM CRYSTAL'S STORY

- For many people, overcoming the stigma and lies from the *War on Drugs*, is an uphill battle we face in educating ourselves about healing through these psychedelic medicines.
- These psychedelic medicines – at the right dosage – have the ability to cut through the ego and get to the core of the trauma, essentially achieving what might otherwise take years in traditional talk therapy.
- When feeling panic or anxiety during a journey, it's important to have a plan to calm yourself – also another reason to have a sober partner, tripsitter, or facilitator, who can help you through the rough spots.
- No one really talks about it, but when planning your setting, you should have clear access to a bathroom – both for urinating and possible purging.

CHAPTER SEVEN

Healing Story #3
Freedom. Liberation... Rebirth

STORYTELLER: Ranga, Male, Indian/BIPOC, Millennial

MEDICINE CONSUMED: LSD

DOSAGE: 150 mcg

FOCUS/GOAL/INTENTION: Observation

BEST PART OF THIS JOURNEY: Seeing things in a completely different light

BIGGEST CHALLENGE OF JOURNEY: So freeing that, paradoxically, it led to some internal doubts

....

PROFOUND HEALING JOURNEY STORY DETAILS

This journey started with consuming the LSD at my house and then eventually going for a 5-mile slow walk, more of a wandering.

In this journey, it was like a rebirth – or being born for the first time. The life I lived before my first psychedelic experience three years prior seems like it wasn't me. All these questions arose from my actual childhood, but I had no conscious memory of them. I never realized the baggage I was carrying. The LSD gave me the opportunity to shift my internal reality.

I did not set a specific intention with this LSD journey, but with every subsequent trip after that, I developed this respect for the medicine. LSD wasn't like anything else that could be abused or misused it. It has its own sacred thing going on with it.

This experience was mind-blowing, but it is so hard to put into words; I don't have the vocabulary for it. From another LSD experience (300 mcg) which was outdoors at a beach, I just knew that I was meant to be on that beach and experience what I did. I felt like, yes, this is where my life is heading – and I like it.

I used to have real embarrassment of my body hair and normally can't even remove my t-shirt in public. But about 20 minutes into the journey, I was completely fine with being naked on the beach. So, I am nude, and all these things are happening – and I was just accepting them. I wanted to just be present.

I was able to better understand detachment – from people, things, objects – and I feel like the LSD helped me also see death in a new light. LSD helped me break free from the rigid plans set for me by my culture, society, parents, collective unconscious in general.

I was not prepared for the LSD to push such a hard look at my internal well-being and to put me into a state of complete honesty with myself. I learned life is about having options. I feel life is better.

BIG INSIGHT: I learned I was the one stopping myself – and that information was freeing. Blame is of the past, but responsibility is of the present. It could be anyone's blame, but it is one's responsibility to fix it.

There's always a narrator in our heads, which I don't see as a healthy thing because it often stops us from being a part of the experience. My first experience with LSD was quite shockingly magical in a particular sense because it led me to asking for the first time: Who am I? That question came to existence because I was just wondering if the drug had it me? Am I tripping? Wait, first what's tripping? And what do I mean when I say I am tripping? And it's mind-blowing because there are no substantial answers to the questions.

Inside the psychedelic zone, when the noise and narration stop, I saw things with new clarity. Like I woke up. I noticed a tree standing outside my balcony for the first time.

I am carrying this baggage from my past life, which acts as lenses, which obscures the picture of what I am seeing right now. So, it makes me more judgmental, right? There are reasons that we have stereotypes. So, how do we overcome seeing things with clouded lenses? Because once the psychedelic wears off, you are almost back to the same old habit pattern which is acting out of conditioned mind and not present moment awareness. This is where I met vipassana, a Buddhist meditation technique.

There are two words in the language of pali (language in India during the time of Gautama the Buddha): sañña and pañña. Sañña means perception – and perception is always clouded by what we have learned and experienced. But, once we learn to start coming to the present moment and learn to be equanimous to life events, the sañña becomes pañña, which means wisdom – now being able to see things the way they are rather than the way you want things to be. Psychedelics is a glimpse into meditative state. It's a temporary wisdom, which will get lost if there is no post integration.

KEY INSIGHT: It's important to integrate these journeys because if you don't, you may lose the insights you have during the trip and you might end up going back to the collection of reactive patterns the identity is. The integration kind of becomes the way of life post psychedelic and life is one giant psychedelic trip for which all you need to do is just pay attention.

I have seen significant changes, as I try and integrate my experiences every day. I am not an experienced meditator, but it is something I am working on. The benefits of meditation are amazing.

Slowly it has come to me that my happiness does not depend on any one thing – from material things, nor people, or events, or validation. It comes from a place of, and it's hard to name, but the Divine. I found genuine happiness for the first time… it feels like a state of joy.

People are not talking as much about LSD as they are about MDMA and psilocybin. Some people see psilocybin as the *Holy Grail* of psychedelics, but there are so many others. LSD has been one hell of a great medicine to put you in a state of introspection.

But it's amazing the conversations that are happening now about these psychedelics and healing… I could not even imagine them happening a few years ago.

I think it's all about becoming so selfish to the point that you're selfishly trying to find yourself. And eventually, you become selfless because there is no self [with ego dissolution]. You can't settle for half-baked answers, you have to be really curious in finding the self.

That said, I think there is one thing all religions have gotten right – and that's the [Golden Rule]: do not do something to someone that you wouldn't do to yourself.

I have found my voice, my community… and confidence in myself.

PERSONAL BACKGROUND

I grew up in the southwest part of India, which has a heavy amount of tradition, culture, and rituals – which are important to my story, because they were restricting me to live a particular way and they were sucking the life out of me. I was also bullied as a child… bullied a lot.

I also grew up in an unhappy home. And I am sorry if I am stereotyping here, but I do believe that more than 50 percent of all marriages in India are completely unsuccessful because of our dogmatic culture. And you grow up in a house with parents fighting, not having harmony. And as a kid, you question these things, but you're afraid to ask the question out loud, to the point that I assumed happiness is just once a month thing and rest of the time you are supposed to live based on fear.

The plan for me was to go obtain my master's degree, then land a job right after I graduate. Shortly after that, it would be time to buy a house and get married and settle down. Then, two or three years later, you need to start having kids. And this plan was set for me. And then you work and work – and then when you are 50 or 60, when you retire, then you can finally look into spirituality and happiness.

What psychedelics did was break these concepts for me and put me in touch with my spiritual self.

My dad still expects me to come out of this "phase" of being a nomad or recluse or monk. But I do not care about looks, I do not care about a career. I do not care about convincing society that I am happy. If I'm happy, then I am happy – I do not need to explain further. But his perception is still like, "why are you going involved with these stupid drugs?"

In India, or at least the part I grew up in, the extended family – the relatives who are there – put pressure on your parents, who in turn, put the pressure on you. And in that one way, I'm lucky because my dad and mom don't have many relatives; and the ones we do have are not that connected.

My first psychedelic experience was after I left India and came to Canada to work on my master's degree. I did have a psilocybin trip. I don't think it was as awakening as my LSD experience. I did have insights yet failed tremendously to incorporate them into my life, but that day was equally liberating. I felt happy for the first time – genuinely happy without that happiness tied to any one thing, such as pleasures derived from future moments.

I have also experimented a bit with DMT. You smoke it – and it is very powerful and fast-acting. And next year, I may sit with Ayahuasca. Right now, I am just researching places in the Amazon jungle, rather than trying to find a center here.

As for the future, I don't really know. I am thinking I may want to facilitate psychedelic trips at some point – not from a financial or job standpoint, but from a place of providing help with the medicine.

FINAL NOTE: When I last visited my family in India and told them about some of my insights and experiences, the response I got was… how long are you going to be doing this, and, it is nice for you, but you still need to do life the way it is defined by the society (career, marriage, family, kids, investment, etc.)

EDITOR'S NOTES:

KEY TAKEAWAYS FROM RANGA'S STORY

- The difference between recreational use and therapeutic use of psychedelics is the setting of clear intentions and having a safe, cozy setting. Preparation is essential for intentional psychedelic experiences/healing.
- While all psychedelics are similar, they also have unique characteristics – and effects, so it's important to find the best one for your needs/healing.
- It's better to start with a gentler psychedelic and/or a lower dose – before delving deeper into the medicines and heavier doses.
- These psychedelic medicines can break through cultural norms and expectations.

CHAPTER EIGHT

Healing Story #5
The Mother's Call: Finding Healing
by Listening to the Call

STORYTELLER: Aditi, Female, BIPOC/Indian, Millennial

MEDICINE CONSUMED: Ayahuasca

DOSAGE: 1 serving (from Shaman)

FOCUS/GOAL/INTENTION: Clear blocks to finishing my book; and self-confidence; and healing my heart.

BEST PART OF THIS JOURNEY: Opportunity to connect with my soul in a sacred way and speak to higher realms and get answers about my path and purpose.

BIGGEST CHALLENGE OF JOURNEY: It was very emotional and I was very sensitive for weeks. It felt like everything was crumbling at times but things were being reorganized. Also post-journey challenges: remembering everything and integrating the insights into practice.

....

PROFOUND HEALING JOURNEY STORY DETAILS

They say when you are meant to do Ayahuasca, you will hear the mother's call. The spirit of the medicine, *Mother Aya*, will call you in. You will start to feel her whispers or simply an inner pull or curiosity toward wanting to try the medicine.

When the medicine calls you in, it means there is healing it can offer you. I was intrigued by Ayahuasca but I wasn't called to it. I had heard of other people having intense experiences which scared me. It was an all-night medicine journey where you have an out-of-body experience, connect to deep parts of your soul, and purge the crap out of yourself. This could be toxins, grief, anger, childhood trauma, and anything that is blocking you from your full potential and whole health.

I imagined it would look like a group of people losing their minds – hysterically crying, puking their brains out, and holding on to any glimmer of reality with desperation.

It was nothing like that for me. My Ayahuasca experience was quite the opposite. It was quiet, and soft, with little to no puking. The facilitators laughed when I told them what I thought it would be like, and they confirmed it can be an intense ceremony sometimes. They explained that each experience was unique and brought us exactly what we needed.

One thing I can say for sure is that the experience was life-changing without a doubt.

To prep for the ceremony, the facilitators encouraged us to eat lightly the day of and to bring fruits for the altar as well as a yoga mat and blanket. From the group of colleagues, 2 of us decided to go.

If my colleague had decided not to go, I definitely would not have gone. The place was hard to find, I did not have service there, and our cab driver did not speak English. But luckily together we were able to find our way there.

The trek was a voyage, but once we got there, it was quite majestic. We were the first two people to arrive. It was a large empty dome inside of a jungle. It had a wooden floor and a net covering the sides to block the bugs from getting in.

We all laid our mats in a circle and the Shaman and her team sat at the front of the dome facing us. This Shaman traveled from Peru, leaving her country for the very first time to bring this sacred medicine to Tulum. Her team had been guided by spirit to come to offer this ceremony here. It was very special to be part of this experience.

Whenever I thought about partaking in Ayahuasca, I always wanted to experience it in Peru – so it felt like the medicine had come to me, directly from Peru. I was no longer scared. I felt like I was exactly where I was supposed to be.

The ceremony started with the team explaining the events for the night, clearing the space, and chanting to help create protection around the dome. Then one by one each of us were invited to have one drink of the Ayahuasca medicine. It was served in a tall shot glass. We were first given one drink to see how it sat with our system and then were permitted to have up to four drinks throughout the night with the last one being at 4 am.

Once everyone took the first drink, we all went back to our yoga mat beds to lie down. It was completely silent and I was surprised at how quiet it was, but closed my eyes and lay down as I waited for the medicine to kick in. In about an hour, I started the feel the medicine.

It felt like I was floating, but also still present. It felt like things were moving around me and I knew that I couldn't get up. I just wanted to curl myself up into my blanket. At times, my mind wandered off into thinking about mundane things like messaging my Airbnb host about something.

Other times it felt like I was having deep revelations, contemplations, and thoughts about my life. There were times I was having full in-depth conversations with myself and sometimes with something bigger than me.

At one point I felt Mother Aya come and talk to me. It was a warm, loving, welcoming presence. A deep love I had never experienced before. *An all-consuming, unconditional deep love.*

I felt touched by her love. She told me that I was on the right track and that I was indeed supposed to write this book about self-care and teach about it. At the time, I had started writing my now-published book, *The Self-Care Habit*, but I was having major doubts and imposter syndrome around it.

I got messages about my childhood, my purpose, and new perspectives and insights about my struggles. So much was coming through that I wished I could've had it all recorded or written down. But I decided to trust that I would remember exactly what I was meant to.

We all had buckets next to us in case we needed to throw up, but not many people used them that night. Maybe two of us. I felt myself wanting to purge at one point but I couldn't get it out. One of the facilitators saw I was struggling and came to help me. She sat next to me as I tried to let it out and told me, you came here for your healing, allow yourself to receive it.

I felt so awkward and uncomfortable at the idea of throwing up in front of everyone, especially when it was so silent. I felt like I was disturbing the peace. The facilitator could sense this and whispered to me, "Think that no one else is in this room but you and me. Receive your healing." Those words were everything for me in that moment.

DEEP INSIGHT: This experience represented an exact replica of how I felt in real life. I held myself back from expressing my full self because I didn't want to rock the boat or cause a scene. I was always told to take the high road, be pleasant, and not create any trouble. But now I was faced with a dilemma, was

I going to disturb the peace and get my healing or let go of my healing to keep the peace in the room?

I decided I wanted my healing and to get what I came for, so I opened myself up to purge. It felt so much better after I did. Soon after the fourth drink was offered, everyone went to sleep and woke up in the morning. We sat in a circle and each shared our experience and the facilitators gave us their reflections as well which were so powerful.

When my turn came, I spoke to the facilitators about the messages I received and they shared with me how Mother Aya teaches self-love and self-care so it wasn't an accident that I was here.

I was blown out of my mind. I had prayed for help with finishing my self-care book, months prior, and Mother Aya directly had called me in. She initiated me, gave me permission, and gave me ideas for my self-care work that I was getting prepared to teach.

The entire experience was magical.

But what happened after was even more magical. They say that psychedelic medicine clears your system of any baggage that is holding you back. And from that clearing, your body emits a clearer signal to the Universe allowing you to bring in what is meant for you.

Within months of the Ayahuasca ceremony, I got promoted at work, experienced a romance that blew my world away, got accepted into a competitive master coach training program, got my self-care book published, and so much more it's insane.

After this medicine ceremony, so many doors opened up for me. It's almost like all of this was waiting for me, but I had to allow myself to receive it and clear the blocks in my way.

Ayahuasca changed my life in more ways than one.

I wasn't looking for the medicine, but I had been praying for a miracle. Having experienced many years of depression, burnout, and dissatisfaction with life, I was always seeking paths to fulfillment. I had come to a place where I was ready for my next level of healing.

In many ways, Ayahuasca healed my broken heart and opened up a new zest for life that I had been desiring for years. It was the most healing experience that I didn't know I needed. I pondered if Mother Aya was actually the one who called me to Tulum.

As I write this story, I have recently moved to Tulum – to be here for a longer period of time. I'm excited to continue to connect with this divine energy, follow my soul's calling, and share it with you.

KEY ADVICE: If you feel the Mother's call, be sure to follow it. It could change your life.

PERSONAL BACKGROUND

Toward the end of my six years in Corporate America, I experienced a low depression, which had me questioning everything. I wondered if this was all the rest of my life was going to look like. Going to work, coming home, doing it again tomorrow, and attending events on the weekend. It felt drab and unpromising – what was the point of it all? During this time, I felt dead inside, was at my highest weight, and was barely making it through the days.

Realizing how much I was sinking, I knew something had to change. I asked my heart what it truly wanted if no one was watching and started to forge a new path. I quit my "safe" job, moved to another city, and started graduate school. This was the beginning of a new chapter and it was also where I went into an even deeper depression and major identity crisis. I didn't know who I was, or where I belonged, and I deeply despised myself for not having the answers when it seemed like others had it all figured out.

As I dragged myself through these years, I started practicing self-care to nurture myself through the wounds. It was the only thing that helped make life a little more bearable. As I did this, I found an opening inside myself. A curiosity, a wondering, a potential for a new possibility.

I started to take bigger risks because my soul knew I couldn't go back to my old life. After graduating with my master's degree in marketing, I launched my own marketing business offering coaching to small business owners. This soon transitioned into life coaching on stress management because that's what we ended up talking about in most of our sessions.

Having experienced my own burnout and depression in Corporate America and business, I was able to relate to my clients and offer them helpful tools. During the pandemic, I was invited to deliver a virtual stress management talk at a billion-dollar company to its employees all over the world. That's when I decided it was time to write a book on how self-care saved my life.

And a year later I found myself in a jungle drinking Ayahuasca.

I met a colleague who lived in Tulum through a company I do life coaching for. She often told us coworkers to come there. I had heard of Tulum being the new hot spot to visit and for digital nomads so I decided to take the leap. Plus having a friend there made it feel safer to try it out.

The week I arrived, I met my coworker for the first time in real life; we had been *Zoom friends* prior. Four of us colleagues met up, who also happened to be in town at the same time Was this a dream come true? I was literally hanging out in another country with my coworkers. Not for a business trip, but an actual meet-up!

Since we all worked in the psychedelic medicine space, we were often sharing news with each other. The next week one of our colleagues shared an opportunity to go to an Ayahuasca ceremony. I hadn't felt the call to do Ayahuasca yet, but I had a feeling I would probably do it in the next 3-4 years.

My colleagues were discussing going and I started to wonder if I should go too. I mean what a sacred opportunity, to do Ayahuasca with my psychedelic family! I didn't want to miss out on this opportunity but I also didn't feel ready. I hadn't felt the call from within.

That week I started to feel Mother Aya calling me in. I heard in my spirit, "come child, come." I wondered if what I felt was real and if this is what it meant to be "called" to the medicine. As the week went by I started to feel less scared and more interested in the possibility of doing Ayahuasca.

By the time Friday came along I decided I was in.

EDITOR'S NOTES:

KEY TAKEAWAYS FROM ADITI'S STORY

- The plant medicines, especially, are known to have the power to call you to a ceremony. You'll suddenly start to see the medicine in news stories, in discussions with friends, in your dreams. And when these medicines call to you, it's specifically for the purpose of healing.
- Of all the psychedelic medicines, Ayahuasca is most known – almost to a surreal level – for purging; and that purging is usually in the form of vomiting… or defecating. But there are indeed other ways to purge the stuff that needs releasing, including yawning, giggling, coughing, crying.
- Ayahuasca, because of the powerful element of DMT in the brew, has a reputation of being a medicine that can take people on gnarly journeys, challenging journeys… but it partly depends on the level of trauma and the amount of healing needed.

- Psychedelic medicines can be life-changing experiences, typically listed among the top experiences in a person's life. These journeys often lead to not only amazing healing, but powerful insights and critical "downloads" of helpful information.

OTHER DETAILS

Aditi is the author of The Self-Care Habit, *an invited speaker, a psychedelic guide, and an intuitive life coach. Learn more about her book here: aditicreative.com/book*

CHAPTER NINE

Healing Story #6
Enough Was Enough

STORYTELLER: Todd, Male, White/Caucasian, Gen X

MEDICINE: MDMA

DOSAGE: 125 mg; booster of 75 mg

FOCUS/GOAL: A fact-finding mission to find out why I couldn't stop hitting the same wall(s).

BEST PART OF JOURNEY: The *Answer*. All of it. Every single bit.

BIGGEST CHALLENGE OF JOURNEY: Everything that comes after it: integration. The journey itself was *Magic*.

....

PROFOUND HEALING JOURNEY STORY DETAILS

I completed this journey in a hotel room, with an eye mask and spa/ambient music in my headphones. Lots of water. Lights off. And my journal. My journal was key. I also wore a sweatshirt with LOVE emblazoned across the front. I was comfortable. I worked with a friend who was well-versed in MDMA and was the perfect guide for my journey – both in prepping me for the experience and for sitting with me during it.

After taking the first dose (the bigger of the two), I closed my eyes and listened to the music. I wasn't sure what to do. When I opened my eyes under the mask, I felt like I was speeding through space. Like *Star Wars*.

When I closed my eyes, I had the POV from a drone flying over a huge estate in the countryside. I saw a man walking in the side door and I buzzed down to see who it was. An Instagram poet that I was friendly with. Jeff was known for his vivid, honest accounts of his life. His failures. His loves. His lies. His fetishes.

All of it.

I'd open my eyes and off through space. Close them and the drone was flying over a different estate in the woods. And there was Jeff again. Walking in the side door. I understood the message: Be open. Be like Jeff.

This went on. Flying through space. Huge mansion and Jeff. I pulled off the mask and journaled what I was seeing and what I believed the message to be. I have no idea how long I had been on my journey, but I felt good about how it was starting.

I took the second dose. And immediately fell asleep. I was pissed. I felt like this journey was my only chance to get an answer and I didn't want to sleep through it. When I woke up – and again with no sense of time – I said to myself, "I don't understand what the fuck I'm doing here. I've had years of therapy. I've done all the work. I've repented for my mistakes. I've forgiven my mom time and time again. What the fuck am I supposed to do?"

And a little boy's voice said, "You need to forgive yourself."

Me: *What the fuck do you mean I need to forgive myself?*

Boy: *When you were seven and that thing happened with your mom – you abandoned me. Now you feel shame every time you're reminded of it.*

Me: *Shame?*

Boy: *Yes, for abandoning me. For abandoning yourself. You never allowed yourself to live your life. You were afraid to rock the boat. You started to ask for permission to live your life and if you didn't get it – you'd live the life others wanted for you. Your parents. Your partners. Your bosses. Forgive yourself.*

I started sobbing and tore off the eye mask. It's me! I need to forgive me! I started writing it over and over and over again, I forgive you. I forgive you. I forgive you. I forgive you. It made so much sense.

I put the eye mask back on and asked the boy, "What do I do after I've forgiven myself." The boy responded, "Well, now you love yourself." Holy shit!

I tore the mask off again and started writing, I forgive you. I love you. I forgive you. I love you. I forgive you. I love you. It was amazing.

Eye mask back on. Now what? And the boy said, "Well, now you get to grow up." And I took a deep breath and was completely still. Now I get to grow up.

After some time, I took my eye mask off and started writing a letter to my wife. I wrote about what I was experiencing and how I now understood that any time I was triggered in shame, I became this 7-year-old boy. I wasn't engaging in the complicated parts of life as an adult. And that likely made her feel 7. How could we possibly engage as adults?

I texted my mom and apologized to her. I explained what I was doing and how I was feeling and how I understood her fears around me for the first time. I said I would write more later. I texted my brother with a similar message. And then I texted my friend and said, "Thank you for saving my life."

I put the eye mask back on and started to explore all the areas of my life. The choices and mistakes I had made. The professional situations that went sideways. Friendships that were lost. The hurts I had caused. Fight. Flight. Freeze. I understood all of it. I could see where the choices came from. I could see how the shame got triggered and the choices were made.

I saw why I struggled with food and my weight. I saw all of it. I understood healing. For the first time. Finally, after six or seven hours, I took off the eye mask and said to my friend, "I want to go outside. I want to see how the world looks through my own eyes for the first time.

The following day, I stayed in the room and wrote and slept and wrote some more. The day after that, Sunday, I flew home. As the plane touched down in Oakland, I texted my friend, "I feel like I have a whole new operating system, but the world is still the same. What do I do now?"

He texted back, "Oh, that's called Integration." What the fuck is Integration? I had a decoder ring to my life now. I knew what it meant when I felt dark or sad. That boy was telling me he was scared. So, I could scan a scene and look for what was scary and tell him/tell me that all was okay.

Still, the world was the same. I felt like I was seeing everything with IMAX clarity while most people were still sleepwalking. I was already a feeler. This was nearly unbearable. So, I started studying Integration. I joined an online community. I went into Integration Circles. I leveled up my meditating. My journaling.

WARNING ADVICE: I made the mistake of shouting from rooftops about MDMA during a time when I should have been quiet. It's taken all of every day to find the peace I have now. Integration is a practice. It's daily. It's ongoing. And it's forever.

I'm grateful every time I find myself responding in alignment to things that used to cause me to react out of control. Still...I don't always get it right and I have lots and lots of work to do.

This journey is among the most important experiences of my life. I won't compare it to getting married or becoming a father. It's different than that. But it's everything.

I will continue to use psychedelics therapeutically and have. I've since used psilocybin and have had a microdosing practice (off and on). I've also used small doses of Ketamine and have found the message I get during those short journeys to be profound. I suspect I will do more of both.

KEY TAKEAWAY: Intention. Intention. Intention. Know what you're looking for. Be clear. Be kind. Set & Setting is everything. Mostly, though, have a DEEP understanding of Integration. KNOW that the journey is the start. Not the end.

PERSONAL BACKGROUND

I was raised in an upper-middle-class life. Totally normal. Played sports. I was a good athlete and soccer was my best sport. Fit in. But never felt like I belonged. I always felt a little different. As though I saw things and felt things differently.

I have battled with some form of depression for most of my life. I could hide it. Mostly. I think many people would have been surprised by how hard life felt for me. Sometimes I have flashes of that still. I was 13 the first time I thought about taking my life. I wrote two suicide notes. One much later. 20 pages. Still the most authentic thing I've ever written, maybe. But, I could never do it. I would never do it. I just didn't want to be alive. I didn't want to die.

I felt connected to the Universe and Energy before I had any clue what that meant, but I was also a sarcastic asshole. I didn't let people get close to me – even if they thought they were. I was deeply bonded to animals.

I have an older brother, but we weren't terribly close. He was and is brilliant. We're closer now. My parents split when I was 19, but had no business being married. My mom was a teacher. My dad a public defender. I'm closer to my parents now than I've been in a long time.

But my healing journey was spurred by an April 2021 trip when I went to visit my mom with my son. My brother was going to be in town with one of his boys. My relationship with my mom is complicated and grew more complicated by the year.

I've had plenty of therapy. And still... So, I told my son, brother, and nephew that this time it was going to be different. I was going to get along with her. But...as soon as I walked in the door and saw her, my entire body seized (more than it ever had before), and for the next 48/72 hours, I was as mean or meaner to my mom than I had ever been.

I knew I had to do something. I told a friend that I was looking into trauma therapy. Hypnosis. Perhaps I had been molested. Something. Anything. I needed to find out because it just didn't make sense to me. Why, after all these years and after all the therapy, was I still running up against the same walls?

I wasn't suicidal, but I didn't want to be alive. My friend forwarded me an article about MDMA therapy and I knew what I needed to do.

EDITOR'S NOTES:

KEY TAKEAWAYS FROM TODD'S STORY

- Psychedelic medicines allow for unconditional love and unconditional forgiveness – of others and ourselves.
- During a psychedelic journey, your sense of time is usually completely disconnected from reality.
- Introspection and reflection of past decisions, relationships, experiences, etc., is a common occurrence in a psychedelic journey.
- Most experts warn people who participate in psychedelic journeys to not make any major decisions while under the influence of the medicine – and that includes texting people.
- When people experience trauma in their lives (and we all have, in some form), all sorts of things can trigger a negative response – people, words, places, smells, etc. Psychedelic medicines get to the heart of trauma and remove or reduce those triggers.

CHAPTER TEN

Healing Story #7
Circling Death & Dropping into the Womb

STORYTELLER: Jessica, Female, White/Caucasian, Millennial

MEDICINE Consumed: Ayahuasca

DOSAGE: 2 servings

FOCUS/GOAL/INTENTION: Merge me with my Soul at all costs/heal parental wounds

BEST PART OF THIS JOURNEY: Facing fear head on and understanding more of my parents' pregnancy journey.

BIGGEST CHALLENGE OF JOURNEY: Choosing to die each "round" of death.

....

PROFOUND HEALING JOURNEY STORY DETAILS

I was called to Ayahuasca in May of 2021 and sat with Mama Aya that following November. I had been on a DEEP inner child healing journey for a year and a half leading up to this experience. I knew I had reached a ceiling with talk therapy and I needed help with subconscious reprogramming. Aya found me at a pivotal turning point in my life. I was in the midst of transforming ALL of my relationships with people, my work, and my home at the time. Aya carried me over the finish line.

I watched as many YouTube testimonials from people who sat with the medicine. I came across a particular healing center located in Costa Rica several times, and found that I knew people who attended it. I followed the signs and booked my retreat with them. They prepare you in advance with diet, medication weening expectations, and they provide a ROBUST experience while in their care.

I was emotionally, physically, and mentally on empty when I walked into the center – with hope in my heart carrying me into the retreat.

On the first night of medicine, Mother Aya showed me all my patterning that was holding me back at the moment. It was very clear, yet gentle.

On my second medicine day, while integrating the journey from the night before, I heard the voice in my head letting me know that on this night I would face death. It wasn't ominous or scary, it was an intuitive knowing. I was calm entering the Maloča that night, unlike the night before when I started crying outside the Maloča before I even entered!

This night I was anchored and centered. Rythmia provides you with intentions that you can use for your journeys. This night my intention was to merge me with my soul at all costs. After my first cup of the medicine, I went into my meditative state, breathing and preparing my body and mind for what was to come. It was a struggle to get off the mattress to get my second cup, and I had to bring my bucket with me. I was sure I was going to purge while waiting for my second cup, but I also knew the second cup was going to take me where I needed to go.

I finally made it up to the altar where a female shaman gave me my second cup. I drank half and had to choke back my purge. I was able to finish the second half and received assistance getting back to my bed. I don't know how long I lasted, but I tried to keep the medicine in me for as long as I could. I felt myself beginning to leave this place while I put my head deep in my bucket. The purging began and the helpers gathered around me.

This is when I slipped from this reality into wherever I went. I could hear what was happening around me start to fade away and the voice inside my head said "it's time to lay down now." I laid down, felt my body involuntarily taking a deep inhale and hold my mouth shut. I was dying. I slipped fully away and was greeted by my deceased grandmother (Maam). She was dressed up, walked me to an entryway and introduced me. She said "this is my granddaughter, she's always prepared!" Then let me know that she could not go with me.

I entered what felt like several circles of death. It was all energy, colors, sounds, feelings. It's hard to describe; it wasn't a visual experience, but more of a sentient experience. Each circle of death required me to release something I heavily identified with in my waking life. Perfectionism, unhealthy coping mechanisms, the lies I told myself, the walls I built around me, my deepest insecurities and fears, everything I've avoided and things that I believed were true that were built on lies and trauma.

During one of the circles, I could hear guttural screaming. I realized it was my ego, me, the human Jessica. The screaming was coming from inside the house, though in retrospect, it was someone in the Maloča screaming, contributing to my experience. But everything that happens in the Maloča is part of your experience.

I struggled to push past the final rounds of releasing my human identity. We had been advised that when things became too overwhelming to come back to our breath and remember that the universe rewards bravery. The irony here is that, when I died on the mattress that night it was from suffocation. (Or what felt like it.) I was trying so desperately to move past where I was to fully die.

The sounds of hissing and sinister laughter were terrifying. I started trying to get back to my human memory to remember something that could help me push past this stretch. The sentiment of 'the Universe rewards bravery' came flashing before me and I was immediately blasted through death. I became energy. Through that portal I was met by my father with angel wings and we spent some time flying around the cosmos.

A voice came in and told me that my time was up and that I had to continue on my journey. I accepted that and dropped into a very tight and warm container. I could feel the tightness around my shoulders and arms squeezing me into a ball. I could barely move. I had been dropped into my mother's womb. While in utero, I witnessed the programming of my nervous system and re-experienced my birth!

The death and rebirth journey, as terrifying and difficult as it was, brought color back into my life again. I was grateful again. I loved the grass again. Seeing stars wowed me again. Seeing clouds would bring me a smile. It helps put things in perspective in terms of self-limiting beliefs, stories I was telling myself that were not serving me and were only holding me back.

I was able to leave a bit of my fear in the other realm and come back to this one with a cleaner slate.

Integration was a challenge at first. I did not sign up for the integration package the center offers. I scoured Spotify for a podcast related to Ayahuasca integration and after I burned through those, I moved onto general psychedelic integration podcasts and episodes. In January 2022, I found in an integration therapist and in May of 2022 I found my support community (Empathic Health).

All of these resources helped me feel less alone, helped me expand on my understanding of the healing process, navigate the expansions, and appreciate the beautiful life that I have been gifted.

I strongly recommend finding an integration support therapist or community before embarking on any psychedelic journey.

FINAL THOUGHTS: This was my most significant life-changing experience. I have such a greater appreciation for the small things, life as I know it, and a zoomed-out perspective of what really matters and what doesn't. Since this journey I've had two psilocybin ceremonies and the occasional microdosing experience. I left my corporate life and I'm fully immersed in the world of healing and psychedelics as a career now. I believe that sharing our experiences might help others be called to their journey toward healing too.

PERSONAL BACKGROUND

I grew up on Long Island in a lower-middle-class town with blue-collar parents.

I've always struggled with anxiety since I was a child and I've experienced severe bouts of depression in my 20s and 30s. And my quest for healing and transformation is really rooted in trying to mend the wounds that I had ignored from childhood, which were playing a role in my romantic partner choices.

I turned to healing so that I could find out why I was choosing romantic partners that did not meet my needs, in hopes of ending the toxic cycles I was playing out repeatedly.

Before psychedelics I was prescribed a generic brand of Lexapro. I weaned off of that before my retreat and I have not gone back to any pharmaceutical medication since.

EDITOR'S NOTES:

KEY TAKEAWAYS FROM JESSICA'S STORY

- These psychedelic medicines are able to help clear away old baggage so that you can experience life and the world in new and profound ways.

- One of the most agreed-upon elements within psychedelics – and especially plant medicines – is that people get called to work with the medicine. We should not be seeking or chasing these medicines; when you're ready for it, the medicine finds you.

- The medicine will always show you what you need to see/do/experience – as long as you fully surrender to the medicine.

- At higher doses of these medicines, people experience "death." Not physical death, of course, but ego death/dissolution, though it may feel a bit like you are dying.

- One of the big themes in healing – including healing using psyche-delic medicines – is healing the inner (wounded) child. These wounds from childhood – being abused or mistreated, feeling ignored or rejected, suffering feelings of neglect or being unsafe – are often deep and painful, and need to be cleared so that we can have a healthier view of ourselves and the world around us.

CHAPTER ELEVEN

Healing Story #8
The Bullshit Machine That is Me:
Releasing My Addiction

STORYTELLER: Guy, Male, White/Caucasian/Mixed Race, Baby Boomer

MEDICINE CONSUMED: Dried psilocybe cubensis (Magic Mushrooms)

DOSAGE: 3.5 grams

FOCUS/GOAL/INTENTION: Consulting with the Sacred Mushroom
about what's next

BEST PART OF THIS JOURNEY: The PURGE

BIGGEST CHALLENGE OF JOURNEY: The PURGE

....

PROFOUND HEALING JOURNEY STORY DETAILS

I stare into the rushing current of the emerald-green river. My eyes fix on the chaos of the turbulent waters, while each ray from the hot, summer sun fractures into an electric shattering of light across the powerful flow.

Closing my eyes and inhaling long and deep, my prana dances up my spine in its own sparkling display. A long slow exhale aligns my energy with the flow of the beautiful river before me and I bring my hands together in gratitude for just being.

The previous night was a long one. I had decided to consult with the mushroom about "What was next?"

Having been up in my cabin in the woods for a year now, I left the city after living in an urban environment for nearly 40 years. The draw into nature was an incredible force, one which I didn't fully understand, but followed without question initially.

Then every couple of months after moving up here, I began to question the sanity of it all and consulted with the mushroom – and through this process, something was then invariably revealed or resolved. "What was next" is a common intention for my entheogenic journeys, as the question itself is a sort of statement of surrender to the pending non-ordinary state of consciousness.

KEY ADVICE: With the Sacred Mushroom, the more your body, mind, and spirit are in stillness and surrender to the experience, the more profound and beneficial the outcomes. The mushroom knows what's best for you and their ageless wisdom delivers loving insight direct from the *Collective Consciousness*.

After fasting for the day, I made a Lemon Tek tea with 3.5 grams of dried psilocybe cubensis, which is on the high side of a medium dose for me. I took some Rapeh and puffed on a cigarette of nicotina rustica to cleanse and strengthen my being for the experience about to get underway, then thanked the mushrooms for their love and guidance and knocked back the tea in a few chunky gulps.

After lying down, I began a body awareness meditation – focusing points of relaxation and awareness in my hands, feet, and jaw – which I've found to be very effective in getting into the 'floating state' of being with a completely quiet mind. It's my favorite place in the world, and a perfect runway to the Mushroom Consciousness.

As the medicine came up, I felt myself slipping away and the mycelium taking the wheel – gently breathing into the entheogenic trance-like experience gradually obfuscated this consensus reality and before long I was definitely not running the show.

I felt the purging bubbling up from deep inside me, a common theme in my mushroom journeys, and an indicator there was energy clearing taking place, and that this wasn't going to be a journey of iridescent unicorns and undulating rainbows. This was going to be work.

When I purge in the *Mushroom Consciousness*, there's no vomit, but what comes out is much more damaging and debilitating than a bowlful of Kung Pao chicken left out in the sun all day. With a massive heave, a long-time addiction exploded in a forceful wretch.

It had come up in mushroom journeys before, but I chose to ignore their message. This time the mycelium was going to win – as was I. I don't know how long I purged for, but I will never forget the force it took to release the addiction that no longer served me.

Like a surgical procedure, the Sacred Mushroom delivered "What was next." And after the blockage was taken care of, I came back into a semi-lucid state, enough to feel the healing that had just occurred and break into gasping sobs of gratitude, while being wrapped in unconditional love.

As the medicine wore off, I was able to process what had just happened. I thought about the lies I told myself in order to keep up a practice that I knew damn well wasn't good for me.

Mushrooms are very good at truth and very adept at putting things bluntly, with love, and often framed with sharp wit. This time around they thought it fitting to give my ego a tagline, as if the Mushroom morphed into the persona of some sassy junior copywriter at a Madison Avenue advertising agency.

"The Bullshit Machine That Is Me," they pronounced. I burst into uncontrollable laughter, repeating the phrase over and over, each time sounding funnier than the last. *Guy, party of one!*

The rushing river darkens as the sun slips behind the deep blue mountains. As I walk back to the cabin in the dwindling light, I meditate on the transformation that had taken place and a wide smile blooms in the cooling evening air. Such a gift.

As each day passed, I continued to feel gratitude – not just for the healing but for just being, and each breath miraculously powering this crazy state of Consciousness we call being human. Around me, the mosaic of nature, a treasure of wonder and creation with no bounds continues to hum her symphony of life.

And me? That addiction is gone, like it never existed – and each day I'm trying my best not to be a bullshit machine. I'll continue to do the work – meditation, mindfulness practices, working with nature, writing, making art, and periodically connecting with our plant and fungi teachers. For me, these are acts in honor of Consciousness and a celebration of the engine of love that powers creation. If that's not living a life of purpose, I don't know what is.

PERSONAL BACKGROUND

I first experimented with psychedelics when I was 14 years old. I think I did it back then as a means of numbing pain, fitting in, alleviating boredom, or just escaping the predicament of puberty [CHECK ALL THAT APPLY]. By the time I was 16 years old, I was no stranger to cannabis, psilocybin mushrooms, LSD, or MDMA.

It's no surprise that this non-intentional, recreational use didn't produce any epiphanies or breakthroughs into higher states of awareness, but it did its job keeping me under the radar throughout the many traumas of high school years.

My story of trauma starts with my father getting killed when I was 12; the helicopter he was flying blew up in a hot summer sky. A few years later, my mother was murdered in her home – stabbed 27 times by someone who was never convicted of the crime but now is dead, as is the cold case around her slaughter. Guess we'll never really know. My sister died a few years later from complications of alcoholism at way too young of an age.

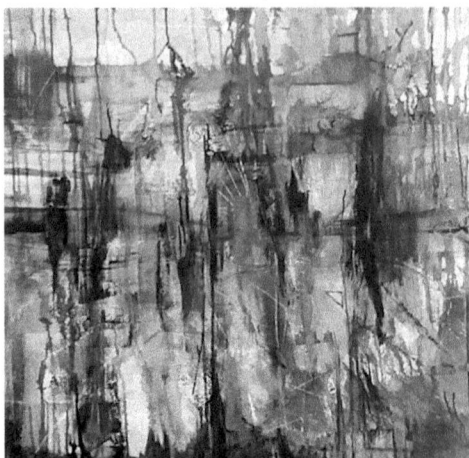

"Morning Garden" 122cm x 91cm Mixed Media on Canvas - Guy Borgford 2020

Being bullied, and never feeling like I really fit in. Being ashamed of who I was on so many levels. And this doesn't even consider the volumes of epigenetic trauma packed away in my DNA.

And so I sealed the pain and numbed myself for decades.

And according to me, I was absolutely fine – more fine than most people I knew. In my youth I turned to cannabis, alcohol, and a host of psychedelics to try and escape the invisible pain, buried deep within me like a darkened, cursed tomb.

I didn't know that with the exception of alcohol, many of these escapes would eventually prove to be the paths directly into healing that which I had always dreaded.

KEY INSIGHT: The stories we tell ourselves and the lies that become truths – what demons can be manifested from our shadows? Trauma lives there – back in the darkness of our self, weaving its many ways and putting our poor little egos into overdrive with its lies.

Throughout my life, I continued consuming a variety of consciousness–altering substances and although gratefully never developed any serious substance abuse issues, I admit walking the line at several points in my life, while always managing to function, while maintaining an aura of control. Control? Yeah, right.

EDITOR'S NOTES:
KEY TAKEAWAYS FROM GUY'S STORY

- Setting an "open" intention (especially tied to surrendering to the medicine) allows the medicine to show you what most needs healing.
- Many people incorporate sacred rituals (especially with the plant medicines) when consuming these psychedelics; these rituals often help with the set and setting.
- Mediation (and other relaxation techniques) is often added to the mix as a tool for calming the mind and body in preparation for the journey from the medicine.
- Sadly, many people attempt to numb their pain (often from hidden/subconscious traumas) with alcohol and other recreational drugs; happily, these psychedelic medicines show great promise in stopping these addictions.

....

Ode to Aya
by Guy Borgford

That sound of present joy
The voice of love
She has no beginning
She has no end
She is everything and everyone
Who was, is, and ever will be.
She is infinite in her love
And divine in her creation
She is the darkness
That cradles the stars

Caressing secrets of the worlds
Beyond ours.
She is the darkness
Of our fears
That keep us from
Our true selves
She is the light
That fills our hearts
Connecting us to eternity.

The warmth of the sun
The crest of the moon
Falling in love
Falling from grace
She is the light, the dark
Always nurturing
Guiding us
Teaching us.
Gratitude is our key
The pass to her magnificence
Surrender is our vehicle
To the unlimited wonders
Of her universal love.
Every breath
Every being
Every drop of rain
Every kiss of the wind
Is her gift
Surrender
Give thanks.

CHAPTER TWELVE

Healing Story #9
The End of Suffering from Depression & Anxiety

STORYTELLER: Urja, Female, Indian-born/Brown/BIPOC, Gen Z

MEDICINE CONSUMED: LSD

DOSAGE: 200 mcg

FOCUS/GOAL/INTENTION: Healing

BEST PART OF THIS JOURNEY: The end of years and years of suffering

BIGGEST CHALLENGE OF JOURNEY: Fear, but surrendered to it

PROFOUND HEALING JOURNEY STORY DETAILS

I was diagnosed with chronic anxiety, depression, and trauma. Speaking in layman's terms, I was suffering a lot. I had thoughts of suicide… things seemed like they would be easier if I just ended it.

You know the point when it's too much? There is a correlation between suffering and break out. I got to the point where I could not take my suffering any longer.

I decided to take this healing medicine LSD in an attempt to end my suffering. I had heard about psychedelics and their healing stories but was living in too much fear to try them… until now.

LSD changed my life. It showed me my calling and what this life is all about. It felt like I laughed and breathed for the very first time.

As the onset of the medicine began, I remember how my eyes filled with tears regarding a great appreciation for this beauty that surrounds us.

REALIZATION: Years and years of suffering broken down one night by this beautiful medicine, LSD. It taught me much more about the human psyche than 6 years of doing traditional psychotherapy had.

How was I sleeping for so long? Had I just been born? All my concepts, all the barriers started melting down, which showed me how these concepts and structures only block us from living happily. I had a total ego dissolution, and the entire universe, every manifest form merged into one.

I was mesmerized by this creation and had a profound appreciation toward everything around me. For the very first time in my life, I understood the meaning of this line from my favorite song by Pink Floyd, "I am you, and what I see is me."

When we are truly able to see that we are one, then we would never want to hurt another.

At this very point, with no egoic identity, no concepts, I understood what it meant to be one, and that how our consciousness is united. Ignorance divides it. This itself gave me peace and most of my healing happened in this space. I was able to forgive a lot of people.

LSD is like a prescription lens. You choose your own lens and that's the perspective you see the world through. I was able to look at the same stuff through various perspectives and each realization drew me to the same very point. **Love.**

We are loving awareness, and our only purpose is to be in this present moment. LSD showed me most of my misery and suffering arose from either carrying the past baggage or thinking about the future and constantly planning. Depression comes from feeling stuck in the past, and anxiety comes from overthinking about the future. However, at that moment time doesn't exist.

I was able to realize what it means to just "be". One of the biggest things I looked at was death. Death of my dog, my partner, my loved ones, myself. There is this deeper realization what it means to die.

A lot of my fear with respect to authority, patriarchy, and death just melted down.

My old defense mechanisms were suppression and denial. On this journey, everything was able to surface, and I was able to unwrap my subconscious mind.

One of the biggest challenges for my trip was when I started to come up from the journey, I literally saw the barriers and concepts coming up. It felt like a prison behind concepts. Concepts of marriage, having a defined life, successful career, these things are structure that society defines.

My journey was to break out of these expectations, and so called "life-book." Watching the barriers come up, I knew the actual work lies in front of me. I only got a glimpse of what it means to be free, what it means to be one. I was able to stop the chasing.

Surrender, surrender, surrender. What does it mean to surrender? As I was coming up, I saw myself fall into a challenging time – so-called fear. I did not know what the fear was. But that's when an insight came to stop fighting it, and just be. I took a few deep breaths, and just surrendered.

Surrender is one of the most beautiful life practices one can learn because we are truly not in control of anything. When humans think we run the world, I believe it's just an illusion.

When we truly understand the infinite that we are, and through LSD I was able to see this, it puts you in touch with God or the Divine Being. The only way I could see was kindness, help where you can, and be here and now.

After my trip, I saw how the habit patterns and ignorance comes right back up, so I went for a 10-Day Vipassana Meditation as part of my integration. I knew the peak would not last, and there are many people who have experienced an altered state of consciousness through meditation.

I am a beginner meditator, but I have seen peaks of "oneness" during meditation. By focusing on sensations, and remaining equanimous to it, we stop the habit of reaction. Wisdom starts arising when we truly observe and not react. It will start changing. If we look into this grand unfolding of the cosmic evolution, we will see that nothing lasts. With this insight, when we remain equanimous and stop the habit pattern of desire and craving, and aversion, we truly begin to taste the sweetness of life.

Since my spiritual journey, I have experienced other journeys with LSD, Psilocybin, DMT, and MiPT (methylisopropyltryptamine, a lesser-psychedelic substance of the tryptamine class). Each psychedelic substance opens a new realm of consciousness; however, the message always remains the same: Be here now – in the present. The minute life starts getting complicated, I know I am reacting to something. But the reality of present moment awareness grounds me.

My companion in this journey has been my partner, who has kept me grounded and that gives me lots of confidence when doubts arise. After my experiences, I started being more honest with my family.

All of these experiences have been challenging, but it's not our job to change anyone. We absolutely can show the path, but not walk the path. I am very thankful to people like Ram Dass, Alan Watts, Terrence Mckenna, The Shulgins, Jidhu Krishnamurthi, Osho, SN Goenka for being my spiritual teachers.

I am now on my path and will continue having experiences with different psychedelics and I hope to help people with any kind of depression, anxiety, sexual trauma, or PTSD to overcome their fears and live this life for what it's supposed to be.

PERSONAL BACKGROUND

My upbringing was quite authoritative. I was raised by my parents until 12, and then moved away with my guardians after that. The intention was in a good place, however my anxiety started then.

Living in an authoritative home, where I was not allowed to raise my voice/talk back or form arguments led to a life filled with fear. My depression had begun much earlier though when I saw a lot of fights in the family. Not having a defense mechanism or ability to cope, watching suffering all around me made me prone to avoiding conflicts later in life, living in constant fear.

One of the biggest triggers for me was sexual trauma by relatives that I had experienced twice at the age of 10 and 14. After such incidents I started living in doubt.

I was told family (and relatives) are everything, but my experience was rather negative, including: filled with hatred, fights, and sexual abuse. I always assumed somehow it was my fault, and I never talked about it. Living in fear of patriarchy, I thought I would be hurt by the elders if I spoke about my sexual abuse.

So, to sum it up, unhappy home, financial struggles, angry men, constant fights with my aunt, and subtle intimidation that led me to make drastic choices which just enlarged my own bubble of suffering.

There were a lot of moments where I thought it would be easier if I just were to end it all. There were pre-attempts, but living in so much fear, there was also a lot of fear of death.

I left India to pursue higher education in engineering, which I deeply despised… but continued because of fear of bringing shame upon my guardians, who were financially investing in me. I did not want to be a failed investment for them, nevertheless I turned out to be one, just more confidently after my psychedelic experience.

I get it now. As the famous saying goes: "Trauma passes down. Hurt people hurt people".

My choices in relationships were "toxic." Broken relationships with partners and friends, I always found myself back in the same hole that I started from, just digging deeper each time. At this point in my life, the only thing keeping alive was my dog, Ollie. He was also the very reason I would witness moments of peace and happiness, but it was as fleeting as shooting stars.

Thank goodness for psychedelic medicines, and especially LSD.

BIGGEST REALIZATION FROM PARTAKING IN PSYCHEDELIC MEDI-CINES: Each experience with a psychedelic medicine has healed parts of me that were suppressed by childhood trauma and sexual abuse.

EDITOR'S NOTES:

KEY TAKEAWAYS FROM URJA'S STORY

- Never let fear win. The brain (and ego) may try to raise anxieties and fears, but it's best to simply surrender to them so that you can have a path to healing.

- While you'll see this topic mentioned multiple times, many people experience dramatic breakthroughs when taking a psychedelic medicine – breakthroughs never experienced even after years (or decades) of counseling/talk-therapy.

- People often feel a rebirth after a psychedelic journey – born into a new and beautiful (and connected) life.

- As with psychedelics, life is about surrendering; we think we rule the world, but it's an illusion.

CHAPTER THIRTEEN

Healing Story #10
Self-Inquiry… and Dealing With My Shadow Self

STORYTELLER: Jason, Male, White/Caucasian, Millennial

MEDICINE CONSUMED: Mescaline via San Pedro/Huachuma

DOSAGE: Heroic (approx. 120 grams of dehydrated powdered, mixed in water)

FOCUS/GOAL/INTENTION: Discover consciousness; who is the person/creator/generator of thought

BEST PART OF THIS JOURNEY: Surrendering and embodying pain

BIGGEST CHALLENGE OF JOURNEY: Seeing shadow (negative) side of myself

··

PROFOUND HEALING JOURNEY STORY DETAILS

I chose San Pedro because I discovered, through the power of the medicine itself, that San Pedro really works for me. It really brings me into my body. (More details in the background section.)

I decided on such a high dosage because I did have previous experience with the medicine and I really felt I needed to sit and be with it (no escape), knowing that I would go into a lot of my physical pain and injuries and examining the trauma of the wounded child (since all my physical pain comes from childhood accidents). So much pain at the unconscious level – and the medicine allowed me to observe this – and I was able to be conscious of what had been unconscious… and surrendering to that allowed me to understand what is consciousness – for myself.

I was out in nature, sitting, on a beautiful day at a house on a hillside – for at least 8 hours of the journey. I purged quite a bit on his journey: vomiting, flatulating, laughing, crying. I tried to move around a bit during the journey

– and did some stretching and yoga. Integration started as soon as I did the medicine – and though I don't journal, I paint. I have created many mandalas, using symbols and archetypes; the dominant theme from this journey is the sun (symbolizing unbound play) and the inner child.

I took the heroic dosage in two doses, about two hours apart… which led to a 35-hour journey. The key is holding in the dose for at least one hour (not eliminating through purging). The medicine took effect about 30-45 minutes after taking the first dose. My stomach was empty – in a fasting state.

I started feeling the medicine in my body – in my abdomen, my gut, my chest, the back of my head. It was like little lightbulbs going off on different parts of my body to bring awareness and attention to different regions of my body that had been hurt or stressed and dysfunctional.

After about an hour or an hour and a half, I consumed the second dose. After just about 10 minutes, I felt the sensations and magnitude and intensity of the San Pedro… the consciousness of the medicine. From there, it was coming and going in waves, and some waves would be bigger than others; the big waves were hard and uncomfortable… I could feel how dysregulated my nervous system was at the time. It was bringing me to these points so I could surrender to it – all of it. Surrendering to me isn't just surrendering the stuff we want to let go of, but surrendering the stuff we want to hold onto. (Surrendering to everything.)

Joseph Campbell, an American writer, stated we have about 68,000 thoughts per day, with the vast majority (98 percent) of them being negative – and I wanted to discover who was the generator of those thoughts. Who is creating the movement of thought?

About 4-5 hours into the journey, I came to a place where I was observing myself from a third person perspective. I was seeing myself through the lens of my partner, my dad, my friends, my clients – and it was hard to see myself because I consistently saw a lot of shadow side tendencies and aspects that come out when I was trying to come from a place of love; instead, I was coming from a place of wounding (the wounded child), abandonment, hurt. And it was hard for me to accept those parts of myself. And that lasted for hours – looking at myself from a third person perspective.

While I did not like seeing these images for hours, with all this pain and seeing my shadow, I realized I was seeing them so I could come to a place where I could have acceptance and forgiveness. Not just acceptance and forgiveness for myself but acceptance and forgiveness for everyone I have been in a relationship with… even the Divine. Then the images came back. What taught me the difference between half-heartedly doing something and wholeheartedly doing something. So I accepted them again, but this time wholeheartedly.

Overall, I am very appreciative that I was given the opportunity to took this dose. The whole process and experience from that journey – I would not be who I am today if not for it, and of course, processing it – allowing myself the time and space to integrate it. This particular journey was about two years ago… and I am still integrating it. Still very aware of the stuff I saw that are lessons to remember. It allowed me to realize how great a teacher pain is and to have more appreciation for everything I have gone through in life. The journey was hard on me, but it softened my ego so that it was not as responsive to my hurt and seeing the hurt I have caused on others.

I still engage with some San Pedro journeys – about 6-8 times a year – but medium doses (40-50 grams).

Interesting side note: We need to have a good understanding of the mineral content within our body. We are generally mineral-depleted because of our soil content is so depleted. San Pedro depletes sodium, magnesium, potassium, and copper… those are key for us. Best integration you can do is to focus on the minerals your body needs.

PERSONAL BACKGROUND

I used to race motocross (starting at age 5) before turning to road cycling professionally at age 20. Because of these sports, I have had 32 broken bones and 16 concussions where I lost consciousness for some period of time – from 2 minutes to 2 hours. So, a lot of residual traumas that really only caught up with me when I was 19 or 20 years old. I had actually gotten physically sick earlier, around 15, but masked it by taking drugs, cortisone, testosterone, growth hormones, peptides… exhausting and burning out my adrenals.

I was so very sick. I worked with numerous doctors – like 15 or so – and did all sorts of cutting-edge therapies, including stem cell therapy, ketamine therapy, hyperbaric oxygen therapy, and others… and they all failed. I spent so much money.

I spent the time between appointments and therapies to conduct my own research, and luckily came upon someone who is still a mentor, Paul Chek, who ended up being someone who helped me acknowledge the healer I have inside of me – so that I can take responsibility for myself and be spiritually responsible for the energy that I create and manifest… and heal. He has a lot of experience with plant medicines and he is someone who introduced me to the medical realm.

I then went to an Ayahuasca ceremony, thinking it was only going to be Ayahuasca, but it also included San Pedro. When I did the San Pedro, it was a very hard experience for me – even though I had taken a light dose. It was very hard on my body, and I felt a lot of pain… and I said right then, this is my medicine – the medicine I need to work with.

I work from home, so I make sure to give myself plenty of time each morning for self-care… I use that morning for various therapies and working out... things for myself. Every day is preparation.

I also previously had avoided red meat, avoiding fat, butter, salts – the typical plant medicine diet – but I found I need some meats in my diet or my energy levels drops considerably.

EDITOR'S NOTES:

KEY TAKEAWAYS FROM JASON'S STORY

- Integrating the lessons gained during an intentional psychedelic experience is a lifelong process – not something completed in a day, week, month, etc.
- Healing should be all-encompassing, not only taking advantage of mental healing through psychedelic medicines, but also in physical health and wellness, including diet and nutrition.
- Mescaline, while considered heart-opening and a gentler psychedelic, can be a hard medicine for the body, so be prepared for purging in a variety of methods.
- We all have a shadow side; it's something we try hard to push down deeply inside ourselves and hide, but the traumas are real and in a psychedelic experience we need to face our shadow sides and attempt to heal them.
- Integration can be done in a myriad of ways, from journaling to painting, dancing, singing… it's about finding the best method for you to help understand your experiences.
- Believe it or not, because the numbers are staggering, but even noted neuroscientist and philosopher Dr. Deepak Chopra has said that we have between 60,000 to 80,000 thoughts per day.

OTHER DETAILS

Jason Gandzjuk lives in California and runs his own health and wellness company: Integrative Plant Medicine Therapy. Learn more: https://www.specializedhealthandexercise.com/

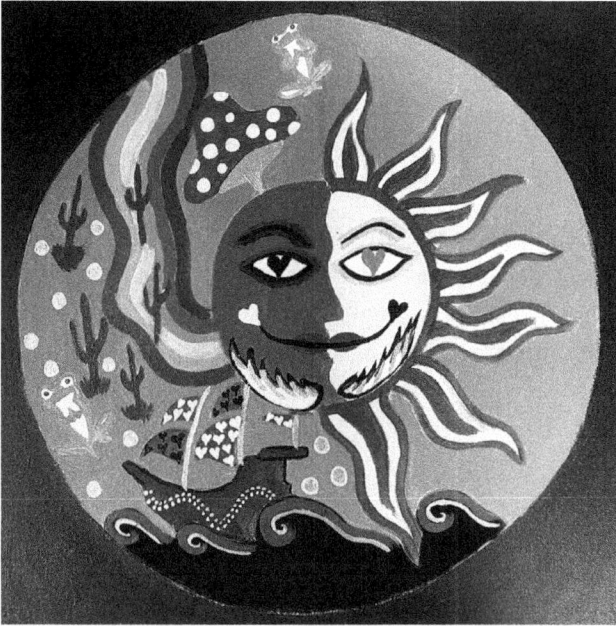

*Mandala created after his Huachuma psychedelic
ceremony, by Jason Gandzjuk.*

CHAPTER FOURTEEN

Healing Story #11
Top of the Pyramid – A 360-Degree View
from the Heart of the Sun

STORYTELLER: Mikaela de la Myco, Female, BIPOC (multi-cultural, first-generation Italian, Afro-Caribbean, and Indigenous Mexican), Millennial

MEDICINE CONSUMED: Psilocybin and MDMA mixed into Cacao, topped with roses and blue lotus

DOSAGE: Psilocybin: 7 grams; booster of 2 grams; MDMA: 100 mg

FOCUS/GOAL/INTENTION: Seeking a download (and purpose) for the next seven years of life

BEST PART OF THIS JOURNEY: Through consciousness, experiencing the meaning of the Mayan calendar day, which was the top of the pyramid in the energy of the sun. The day fell on July 22, the birthday of Maria Sabina and the feast day of Mary Magdalene – and through the journey, I was able to encounter meaning with these important figures. In the minutiae of the everyday grind of being an activist in the psychedelic space, I got to see a much clearer and expanded perspective into what we are all doing this work for – collective liberation.

BIGGEST CHALLENGE OF JOURNEY: A great deal of familial hurt began to arise throughout the journey, and the responsibility came for me to show up for the children my parents were in order to protect them from their own parents' abuse. It was heavy and rather beautiful to be able to do that for them.

PROFOUND HEALING JOURNEY STORY DETAILS

I chose this heroic journey because I was approaching my golden birthday (turning 28 on the 28th) and also entering my Fifth Cycle of life; we change as people (and not just the cells in our bodies) every seven years – and I wanted to see my assignment, my purpose for the next seven years.

According to Rudolf Steiner and other scientists, 7-year cycles are extremely important to doctors, teachers, social scientists, and psychiatrists.

EDITOR'S NOTE: According to Tony Crisp, author of *Every Seven Years You Change*, the Fifth Cycle "is one where the creative process of mind becomes most active. Researchers and inventors seem to make their greatest advances during these years. It is interesting to note that physical science finds evidence of the reason for this in the fact that the association centers of the brain come to their peak efficiency at about thirty-five years of age."

I have been a psilocybin facilitator for the past 7 years, but this journey was my first with other people facilitating and holding space for ME. (I have been a *Mushroom Mother* with a primary focus in holding community and small group spaces, where people can journey through the dark amenta to uncover their ancestor codes, explore and enjoy the body, and heal sexual trauma wounds with mushroom medicine while keeping barriers for entry low.)

I am used to facilitating ceremonial journeys where we sit in a circle with drums and sing and dance. But in this journey, I traveled to Baltimore, to an apartment, with two beautiful facilitators from the Sabina Project, which offers online and in-person Sacred Earth Medicine integration sessions and workshops to inspire radical self-transformation and community liberation, focusing on the BIPOC (Black, Indigenous, *and* People of Color) community.

THE QUEST: It took me several years to build trust – and I believe as a facilitator, you should choose to work with people who are more like friends or rather allies. People you look at and say, wow, I would really be content to make that person's life my own; those people are authentic. So, for me, I had to really know the people who were going to be my guides, who were going to hold space for me – and the invitation actually came from them. That's when I knew it was the right time. It was a peace offering.

Maria Sabina (perhaps the most famous female mushroom healer known; certainly the most famous in Mexico) was known as a visionary, the *priestess of mushrooms, the Mystical Shaman, Wise One, Mazateca curandera (medicine woman)*. Sabina is seen as a saint to some and was one of the most influential artists in psychedelic medicines – and is responsible for the growth of interest in so-called magic mushrooms – for healing and sacred and ceremonial use in the west. She has been a guiding principle in my life, in terms of her humility, artistry, and beauty in journeying.

Before arriving in Baltimore, I also practiced a dieta for a few weeks, really focusing on the food I was eating, but also on my thoughts and demeanor. My goal was on meeting the medicine in a different way – in the purest way possible.

Back to my journey… My facilitators had prepared a mat for me to lie on and played ocean wave sounds while we began our initiatory steps. I was honored that they crafted a special playlist just for me. Masters of their craft. We started with Hapé, a tobacco snuff jungle medicine, to clear the sinuses, remove mucus and prepare the mind for clear vision.

I then drank the medicine. The facilitators gave me special light-emitting glasses and earbuds for the music – and it was like going through a portal of some kind.

After liftoff into my journey, we switched to music playing in the room and eye shades (which I periodically took off). I felt like I was in a dream state… and I had a very inward-focused experience.

So, I went into this journey looking for the download for the next 7 years of my life… and suddenly I was on the top of a Mayan pyramid, looking around with an amazing 360-degree view. I looked down at my forearm, a tattoo of the same pyramid, sun peaking at the apex. A gift from myself of the future into the past for me to later find.

From that top of the pyramid, the heart of the sun, I envisioned a world – a better world – a place where we are working toward something greater… people moving in the proper direction of truth and humility, focused on creating goodness on the planet. Moving toward a shared consciousness filled with hope and joy.

The greatest lesson from the journey was that I am destined to do my work to further this mission over the next 7 years!

Of course, I faced some challenging aspects in my journey. My ancestors were harmed and traumatized in multiple ways during the colonization of our lands. So much trauma from the systemic racism, sexual assaults, and intergenerational abuse at the hands of imperial power and in turn, their families to each other.

Because of these traumas, my grandparents abused alcohol – which affected both of my parents and how they were raised and treated. I was able to visit with my dad's mother – along with my 10-year-old father. I sat with my *little dad* and held his hand while I scolded my grandmother for the way she raised him. My dad passed away years ago and we had a strained – and at the same time – profound relationship, so it was nice to stand with him – and for him.

I also visited with my mom and her family. I wanted to get an apology from that grandmother since in real life (both she and my mom are still alive) she's in denial over the abuse my mother endured at the hands of her husband.

It was definitely challenging, facing and speaking to my relatives.

Toward the end of the journey, I had this strong sense that I needed to stop breastfeeding my toddler. Though I love him and support my son emotionally, I felt it was time to reclaim my body. As my integration, I chose to hold this commitment and hold strong with weaning while still supporting him in all ways.

It is amazing, how the body listens to the cues we give it. As a general notion, when the body realizes it's breastfeeding, it will refrain from becoming pregnant with the intention to maintain nourishment for the mother while she supports her young. When I made this decision to stop breastfeeding, I did not anticipate how quickly my body would cue up the next pregnancy, but it did. And, interestingly, after I did stop breastfeeding, I became pregnant with a little girl who shared her name with me during my experience in Baltimore.

Although my typical dosage is around 3 grams, I know these magic mushrooms can't kill you – no matter how much you consume – so I listened intently to a number that felt right for me and with the encouragement of my guides, aimed higher than maybe I would have before. They absolutely carried me through that portal with grace.

In terms of integrating this experience... we had a sharing circle the next day, and I talked continually with the facilitators until I flew home. I also journaled and drew as much as I could remember. Later in the day, I got a piercing and walked to Edgar Allen Poe's grave – a writer I was fascinated with when I was younger. In the heart of a city like Baltimore, the cemetery was a peaceful and grounding pause.

For balance, I went to a nightclub and danced the night away, walked home, and deeply rested my bones. Even as I recall the details of my experience, I integrate a newly remembered aspect and recall more and more.

The power of telling one's story is so welcome in the integration space and I am grateful for the opportunity to do so.

PERSONAL BACKGROUND

I was a RAVE kid. I think I had MDMA (consumed in the clubs and known as ecstasy) when I was 13. The rave scene was the first place I could feel a connected sense of humanity.

Like many children of the diaspora, I suffered multiple traumas as a child – my own and the intergenerational residue of harm shared from my parents and their parents and beyond.

My greatest wish is that my father could have tried mushrooms as he was transitioning with pancreatic cancer. If I could go back in time, I would give them to him, and in many ways, he does sit with me while I eat the mushroom now.

Though psilocybin has been my primary medicine – whose ceremonial use of mushrooms has worked so well for me and the people I care for, I have also enjoyed the medicines of the mescaline cacti, LSD, and Ayahuasca.

KEY ADVICE: Don't rush into the medicine. Get to know the medicine and the doses which feel comfortable. Facilitators are plenty, we always have a choice. I waited three years for my journey until I felt complete trust with my facilitators. Do your due diligence.

EDITOR'S NOTES:

KEY TAKEAWAYS FROM MIKAELA'S STORY

- While psychedelics remain illegal, it is perhaps even more crucial to work with guides/facilitators/tripsitters that you fully trust.

- Heroic doses of psychedelic medicines are higher than average amounts of the medicine; these journeys are designed for much deeper reflection and healing – and definitely should not be done by beginners, nor alone.

- Psychedelic plant medicines are often consumed in traditional sacred ceremonies (based on long-used Indigenous traditions), but the key is treating the medicine with respect and intention.

- It's wise to be aware that some challenging experiences may occur during a psychedelic journey, but those experiences often lead to the best healing – so surrender to them.

OTHER DETAILS

Mikaela has been led to the ways of sacred intimacy work and the temple arts, Indigenous Mexican ceremony, womb healing facilitation in the ma'at tradition, all under the care of a colorful variety of teachers and guides. She lives in San Diego – occupied Cahuilla and Kumeyaay territory – with her family and friends. Learn more at her website: https://www.mysticjasper.com/

CHAPTER FIFTEEN

Healing Story #12
After Decades of Suffering and Pain,
I Found Love and Acceptance

STORYTELLER: Ariel, Female, Latinx-BIPOC, Baby Boomer

MEDICINE CONSUMED: MDMA

DOSAGE: Initial: 70 mg; booster: 50 mg

FOCUS/GOAL/INTENTION: Spiritual and emotional healing

BEST PART OF THIS JOURNEY: Finding true love and acceptance

BIGGEST CHALLENGE OF JOURNEY: Facing family drama and trauma

....

PROFOUND HEALING JOURNEY STORY DETAILS

I spent a lifetime carefully avoiding and trying to ignore a lot of spiritual and sexual trauma that happened to be in my childhood – resulting in an adult life that was filled with outbursts, crying fits, angry tirades, and railing against religion… and my family.

Psychedelics literally saved my sanity, fundamentally and permanently changing my life for the better.

My life has these dichotomies: the first half a scared and scarred daughter of immigrants, with fears and insecurities, deep scars and anger, and a hatred of my family and religion; and the second half, which I am living now, after consuming psychedelic medicines and taking several journeys, a life of peace, joy, love, forgiveness, and a budding and beautiful spirituality.

My only regret is waiting so long to try psychedelics, but earlier in my life, I never knew about psychedelics – nor were they as available as they have now become.

After doing as much research as I could at the time, the best psychedelic medicine for me – and the one which I could best easily find at the time – was MDMA. I wanted, no, needed, a journey to help find myself, but I was afraid of some of the more powerful psychedelics.

I purposely had a very light breakfast so the medicine would work faster – and I had no other drugs or alcohol for a few days prior, just in case.

I knew with MDMA that setting was especially important, so I prepared a little "trip nest" filled with comfortable pillows with smooth fabrics, cozy blankets, and cool lighting. I also adjusted the temperature in my house to be a bit cooler and made sure I had water and electrolytes nearby. I had my phone with me too, but I wasn't too worried about a challenging trip with MDMA… Still, I wanted to know where my phone was – just in case.

I also decided to use eyeshades to keep me from getting too distracted and headphones connected to an interesting/uplifting mix on Spotify.

My intention for this journey was finding acceptance and self-love, but going into the experience, I had my doubts. Could psychedelics really help me? Wasn't I fundamentally flawed? What right did I have to seek healing? Was God punishing me – or rewarding me?

I took the first capsule and settled into my little nest. Not much seemed to happen for the first hour; I guess I felt a little something changing within and a little energy bubbling to the surface, but nothing more.

So, I decided it was time for the booster pill… and wow, what seemed like just minutes and I was full on into my journey. All of a sudden, my brain was on fire and I was having this crazy download of thoughts and emotions.

I had a few scary moments – not from anything I saw – but the ramp up after the second dose caught me by surprise, both in its speed and velocity… almost like a really strong jolt of electricity to my brain. I had some moments of nausea and a sense of having a full stomach throughout the entire journey.

I had absolutely no sense of time during this journey. I watched with detached interest as the sun moved through the day, but otherwise no idea or interest in time.

I found so much warmth and love and forgiveness. I felt as though this hard shell I had put around me – to protect me from the craziness of my upbringing and to stop any new hurt from affecting me – just absolutely melted… and I almost panicked because it literally felt like the shell was melting and I was worried about the mess I was making, which, of course, was not real.

I was writing so much down during this time. I had so many thoughts and feelings. So many powerful realizations. I wanted to immediately contact some family and friends and share the love, share my revelations, share my joy, share my freedom, share my true self... but whatever part of me that was still somewhat sober suggested I wait until I was done with the medicine.

Amazingly, and so hard to describe, is that I had a long conversation with Jesus about my experiences. He absolutely showed His love of me and for me, and it was absolute; there were not hundreds of conditions for His love, which is how it seemed growing up.

Jesus showed me my place – and value – in the world, in the universe. He showed me that my family and my church were misguided; not evil, but more misinformed and misled... and that information began a slow thawing in my heart.

I know that MDMA floods the brain with feel-good neurotransmitters – and I can honestly say it was the perfect medicine for my journey. I did not want some heavy experience, did not want to see demons or any other challenging visions; I just wanted to experience love – and I did get to experience it (love) in its purest and most amazing form.

To be honest, I kind of got exhausted on this journey. It literally lasted all day and I was happy when I felt the medicine subsiding and my brain and body returning back to normal. My nice little nest was now a bit of a mess – the sign of a long, but truly transformational journey.

Toward the end of the day, I was finally feeling like I could eat something, so I got up and made myself a light, but hearty meal. Before bed, I also took a supplement of 5-HTP to help replenish my serotonin. I had read that with MDMA, there can be a "hangover" the next day because of how much the brain's neurotransmitters get flooded – and exhausted – by MDMA. I also took NAC (N-Acetyl Cysteine), as well as Vitamins C and D and a multivitamin. I also took some magnesium, for sleep.

I have to say that the next day, which I spent mostly recovering, relaxing, reflecting, and writing, was calm and peaceful. I had a slight, dull headache, but certainly not the hangover that may have happened if I did not take the supplements after my journey.

I have done so much journaling and reflecting since that journey... and I have also since then done a few more MDMA journeys to help with some nagging anxiety and other issues. I have to say that I have never felt better in my entire life. I am actually actively looking for a church that fits me and what Jesus told me in that original journey. Time will tell, but I have also come to realize that I do not need a church or priest to have a connection with God, with Jesus, with the Holy Spirit.

I am also still working on my integration and finding more of my people. I know community is important, but I am still coming to terms with who I am and what I believe, and I think I need to do that before I can truly start accepting people into my life – and fully trusting them.

PERSONAL BACKGROUND

I was raised in a very strict, Latino, Evangelical Christian family. We did not have television or any other "evils" produced by those influenced by Satan. Never any alcohol or tobacco – or other drugs in my household… at least not openly used. Yes, there were many hypocrisies.

Personally, I was extremely sheltered and isolated. It was basically school, homework, chores, dinner, Bible study, and bed… then repeat. I was also abused; in the name of Christ and obedience, I was often beaten when I accidentally (or maybe sometimes on purpose) did something against the many house rules… house rules supposedly based on the Bible. I feel my parents were deeply repressed and perhaps deeply depressed – and a little too quick with the harsh punishments.

I never really had any friends because I was not allowed to visit other households (unless they were creepy and lecherous elders of the church) and I never would have ever invited anyone into the crazy/scary that was my house. I acted out – a lot. I didn't know how to express myself as a child, but also had basically been told that children don't have a voice in the household. Life was minimalist, restrictive, fear-based. I don't think I was ever truly sexually abused by any of the elders, but I certainly felt violated almost constantly.

I was given the name Ariel for its supposed significance – and I was supposed to live up to that. In case you are unfamiliar, Ariel is an angel found primarily in Jewish and Christian mysticism. Ariel means *Altar, Light,* or the *Lion of Good.* Ariel is also used in the Bible to refer to Jerusalem.

The one comfort I still take to this day – and especially after psychedelics – is that Ariel is also known as the angel of nature. Interestingly, as with all archangels, Ariel is sometimes depicted in male form; she is, however, more often seen as female. She oversees the protection and healing of animals and plants, as well as the care of the Earth's elements – and THAT is something I can identify with. That is what the MDMA showed me.

Before psychedelics, I had been very estranged from my family. I left them and the church all behind, running away as soon as I could at age 18, and never looking back.

I didn't have my first taste of alcohol until my 30th birthday. I didn't try psychedelics until my 50th birthday.

After psychedelics, I am slowly rebuilding connections with my family. It is hard and slow-going. I have changed greatly while they are still the same, and, sadly, so much hate and fear to this day. But love always wins, right? So, I will keep working at it – but only at my pace and as long as it does not interfere with the profound changes in my life… in my brain and in my heart.

FINAL ADVICE: Don't let an abusive, closed-minded, fear-based, or even "strictly religious" upbringing define who you are today. We do not need to be damaged or living in pain. We can find healing, understanding, forgiveness, love – and even God – through psychedelics.

Finally, an interesting book that helped me more recently with my integration and understanding is Shiva Somodev's book, *Journey into the Heart of Reality: Spiritual Guide to Divine Ecstasy of Self-Realization.*

EDITOR'S NOTES:

KEY TAKEAWAYS FROM ARIEL'S STORY

- It's important to take a deep dive into psychedelics (including the information in this book), conducting enough research so you have confidence in the medicine you choose to assist you in your healing.

- MDMA is perhaps the most heart-opening psychedelic (though mescaline is a close second), and also one of the best for couples or small groups who are looking to deepen their connections and conversations.

- It's never too late, and you're never too old, to obtain insights and healing through the use of psychedelic medicines.

- Preparation is truly essential for ANY intentional healing journey. The better prepared you are, the safer the experience – and preparation starts with researching the medicine and concludes with set & setting on the day of the journey.

- We carry our traumas with us our entire lives, but these psychedelic medicines can help us release their hold on us by safely facing them, acknowledging them, and moving onward.

OTHER DETAILS

One of two paintings, which I have discovered since my MDMA journey, that really speak to me. It helps that the artist, Koichi Sato, labeled his work Ecstasy Journey. *Just seeing the brown faces make me smile.*

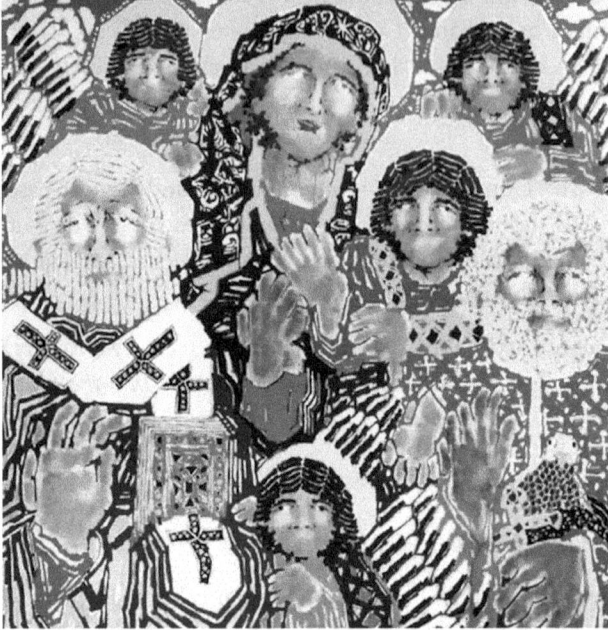

CHAPTER SIXTEEN

Healing Story #13
Reconnecting with Myself; Returning to My Center

STORYTELLER: Alexandra, Female, White/Caucasian/Greek, Millennial

MEDICINE: DMT via Ayahuasca/Yagé

DOSAGE: Several ceremonies; 1-3 shots of the medicine
(dosage controlled by healer)

FOCUS/GOAL/INTENTION: To reconnect with myself after a painful breakup.

BEST PART OF THIS JOURNEY: Oneness. Being part of everything,
an interconnected part of the whole. That I am soil of the Earth where
I came out of and where I will return.

BIGGEST CHALLENGE OF JOURNEY: The whole first day, after everything
began to dissolve and I became aware of how much I have been suppressing
in my body all those years and was afraid to now release (through vomiting or
diarrhea) and even more so, the dark repetitive thought cycles I went down on.

....

EDITOR'S NOTE: While Ayahuasca is the most common name for a psychedelic brew made from the *Banisteriopsis caapi* vine (which is what makes the DMT
orally active) that originated in the Amazon, it is also called different names in
different cultures, including yagé in Columbia and Ecuador, and caapi in Brazil.
That said, all these brews are prepared slightly differently, using different com-
binations of plants. Typically, Columbian yagé uses chaliponga leaves instead of
the more common chacruna leaves in Ayahuasca.

PROFOUND HEALING JOURNEY STORY DETAILS

I had been seeking Ayahuasca/yagé for more than a year when someone referred me to a yagé ceremony that was taking place in Medellin, Colombia, from a family of wonderful Taitas (Cofán tribe).

The ceremonies took place in a beautiful finca (house in a beautiful land) in the woods, in La Estrella. The setting was very homely, warm, sweet, and beautiful. There were many trees and flowers and one very wise cat. The cat was very special to me!

It was a 4-day ceremony, drinking yagé every day. No integration sessions or anything like that.

What was highlighted by the Taitas was the importance of intention. Without setting an intention, we're just tripping and taking the medicine recreationally, and yagé becomes like any other psychedelic. So... my intention was to find who I am after the breakup... and what is my purpose. I was worried – what if the answer will be suffering? (Spoiler alert: It was.)

For each ceremony, we would gather at the maloca at around 10 pm. We didn't start with the medicine until 1 am. It was very dark inside; only a few candles in the maloca. By about 5 am everything would finish.

The first ceremony: After taking my dose of the medicine (smaller than others), I began to question if the medicine was working. But a short time later, the first thing I noticed was the sound of the nature. It was so loud! Next, I would feel warm and cold at the same time. Cold from the air and warm from the blankets. The next thing I knew, my whole body began to dissolve, and I could no longer feel anything from my head down. Or maybe not even my head. I was dissolving and everything was dissolving.

I had no idea of anything (including myself, the world, the Earth, everything I knew including the "I" itself); things began to dissolve, but somehow not disappear. It was becoming one and I could not tell where one thing ended and another one began. I thought, maybe because everything IS one thing.

I lost a sense of ALL. How the world works, why, how it came to be, what it is, what I am, why am I here, how am I here, how the heck am I as I am and what am I supposed to do with and about it. I didn't sign up for anything, it all just happened to me and yet I'm here, a soul in something. A space within another space within another space. This is where we always are, right? In a body, in a house, in a city, and so on and so forth – like the (nesting) babushka dolls.

I HAD NO IDEA OF ANYTHING. I was stripped down of any reference. Even my image, my gender, my name... were not really me anymore... They only seemed like labels attached to me that I was accustomed to using.

I was terrified of purging. Everyone else who had consumed the medicine before was looking forward to this part, but not me. [Purging via vomiting is fairly common when drinking Ayahuasca.]

It was becoming apparent to me that the nausea (in my stomach) and the negative thinking (in my head) were interconnected. It was like one substance split in two entities (mind and body). The instant a negative thought would begin to arise, one that I tend to avoid or suppress in my head, my attention would immediately be drawn to the nausea in my stomach.

I thought I was suppressing only in my mind but it was apparently being suppressed in my body as well. Quite literally, a pile of accumulated intellectual shit was now a physical one, that was taking the form of a horrible stomach ache (one that was making me curl up so to feel it less), a stiffness so present that needed release and I had no idea how to initiate it. I was terrified. Quite literally, I felt like I was full of shit.

Then, my thoughts began to go down on dark thought spirals – which began the challenging part of my journey. I got stuck in repetitive cycles of thought patterns of the exact same thing. Like a mouse on a running wheel. It was torturing to be stuck in the cycles of my negative thoughts.

Three times I interrupted the Taitas – but only when the words would make it out of my mouth, given I was journeying so deeply – to tell him I can't get out of my head, I can't stop thinking.

The next morning, everyone seemed to have woken up happy and connected after the first night. I hadn't. I had spent the night fighting my thoughts, suffering, and crying.

I went to talk to the Taitas, not sure I wanted to do another ceremony. I broke into tears in front of them trying to make it very clear: I WAS TERRIFIED. I wanted to do the second ceremony, but I was trapped in my head and I could not stop thinking. The Taitas said they would give me a small dose for the first cup. Then they would do a healing on me and then I'd have a second cup. (Not that those healings had made any difference in the patterns of my thoughts the night before but as I said, my trust was way too big in the whole process.)

THE SECOND CEREMONY: My new intention for this ceremony was: "Less thinking, more feeling." And to find my strength, my power... as well as the light. What was all that self-hate and darkness that I was so identified with until now? For sure, I have darkness, but I also have light. So, time to find my light, find my strength.

I also thought about what a friend had told me the day prior: "they say one cannot think and breathe at the same time. So… just focus on breathing."

We drank the first cup, and then laid down waiting for the medicine to take effect. As soon as it did, the first thing I did was to breathe – remembering that advice. And I liked that. And then I came to sit and my very first thought was, "Remember that you love yourself, and your love is your power."

After that, from day 3 to day 4, it was becoming better and better. Connecting to the light more and more. Every day was picking up from last.

When I vomited for the first time, as soon as the vomit came out of my mouth and hit the ground it occurred to me that it is soil of the Earth. And so am I. And I was not disgusted by it anymore. It is me and the earth is me and I am it. We are all one. It was going from me to me, back to the earth where I came from and where I will return to.

BIGGEST AND BEST REVELATION: *We are all one. Soil of the Earth. Recyclable.*

I was sitting on the earth, having as much body connection with it as I could, I closed my eyes to meditate and fell into a feeling of being part of everything. The air that is touching my face, I am the air. What is me and what is not me… Me is everything. The cats, the earth, the trees, the vomit… Me was everything.

I also understood why some people call trees the grandparents – "los abuelos" – because many have lived on this Earth before me… civilizations, tribes, philosophers, warriors – and the trees have seen it all; the Earth has so much wisdom that I tear up at the majesty of it all!

I realized that there are such amazing people here! I already feel such deep connection to everybody, and love and understanding, because we are ALL THE SAME. *In a sentence, If I hug you, I hug myself.*

I was even thinking that I'm apparently more hippie than I ever thought I was. It's something that flows out of me, it feels natural… To prefer to stay outside with the earth and the trees as opposed to sit inside the maloca. (I was also annoyed by the music and preferred to listen to the sounds of nature instead.)

The medicine showed me my suffering was coming from thinking.

It also showed me I connected to feeling as part of everything. Just like the flowers, whose purpose is to just be, it occurred to me that our purpose is to be. And so we are (being)!

All our senses are heightened during the journey – because that is who we are. We are senses, we are animals. My soul, my body wanted to go somewhere in nature – and simply carry my mind along as the inevitable but necessary (and tiring) machine that is it. Our minds are machines, and we need to control them is they are useful; otherwise they become useless.

LESSON: Don't think. Just be. Feel. Breathe. Remember that you can do whatever you want! (In fact, this became my mantra: *You can do whatever you want.*

FINAL CEREMONY: My experiences peaked – with the grand finale being the last healing ceremony ending at 5 am – with tears of gratitude!

On that final day, when I was revisiting those negative thoughts (about the breakup), when I was by then already blissful and had purged out all the darkness and accepted what I was earlier, I discovered acceptance. It is not a happy ending (necessarily), but it is an end to the suffering.

I understood that I don't understand (anything), but I am grateful:

- That it is magnificent
- It is huge... vast... massive
- It is ancient
- And I have no idea why and how I came to be and be part of this huge whole thing
- But I am here
- And this was not random
- And for that I am grateful
- It is fucking beautiful
- Wow!

I'm not afraid anymore. Of publishing this. Of it getting to my cousin, to my parents... I have the Truth now. I have and am my own truth and I am an independent entity. I don't need to hide behind parents, stories, and excuses. Whoever understands and whoever doesn't... that's their reality. You get me?

NOTES ON INTEGRATING: As the ceremony was conducted in the traditional Indigenous way, there was no integration after. What I did on my own was to re-read and make sense of my journal entries during the ceremonies, listen to the music to tap back into the experiences – which would bring me to tears and crack my heart open effortlessly every time... and meditate more.

I was teaching yoga at the time so I would invite my insights from yagé into the kinds of things I would share during the yoga classes. I wanted to socialize less and less and spend more time with myself, observing, feeling, contemplating, going deeper.

I kept noticing things as the medicine was still very present inside me.

I wanted to take care of myself like a mother who cares about her child. I started spending a lot more time cooking for myself. And I became aware of the nutrients and foods my body needed, like cheese, dairy, eggs, and good fats like olive and avocado oil. I was more patient with my cooking (while before I would just eat fruit instead of making food), and the flavors-nutrients combination.

I bought Himalayan salt and organic honey. And started instinctively seeking ginger tea after meals for digestion. And I have not thought about my go-to junk food since I have been back. Before, I would think of them every day, but now – no cravings.

MY FINAL CEREMONY SUGGESTIONS: Though my experience is very little, if I may recommend anything to others, it is these two things:

You should ALWAYS have the 2nd cup. (That's when the big realizations and downloads happened for me.) My mantra is "no guts, no story." I recommend that everyone partake in that second cup during these sacred ceremonies; you will not have the breakthroughs you seek without that second cup. That second cup is what gets you to those breakthroughs.

Always go for more than a one-day ceremony – because the experience and insights are cumulative – and the medicine knows when you're there for longer, so try for at least 2-3 ceremonies to get the full benefits.

PERSONAL BACKGROUND

I've been lucky to have parents who allowed me to choose whatever path I wanted to take in life. Even though they are very conventional themselves, I've always been a seeker. I come from a small town in Greece where people follow one specific predictable path and all I ever aspired was anything but that. I wanted to experience life to its core and its depths, to have my perceptions changed by people's stories and wisdom and teachings.

Which is why in the environments I lived, I tried to assimilate as much as possible. To practice religiously during my time in ashrams and yoga schools in India, to learn the language and customs and become part of the culture in South America (mainly in Colombia), to trust and surrender in the hands of shamans, spiritual teachers, and guides.

I started seeking Ayahuasca/yagé after I got dumped by a boyfriend and spent about a month waking up and going to sleep crying, fully disconnected from myself. "This is not me," I was saying to anyone who had met me at that time, constantly sad.

A year before my yagé experience, I had participated in a Jurema (made from the roots of trees in the Mimosoidae subfamily) ceremony, a Colombian plant medicine. For the first time, I talked to myself. I felt that I was always giving myself to other people but never to myself, and what a privilege it was to finally give me to myself, and talk to her. Some of the insights from my experience with Jurema:

As soon as the medicine starting taking effect, I closed my eyes to meditate and thought why would I ever open my eyes... As in, it's so nice here!

After the day of the ceremony, I felt very inclined to spend a lot of time alone. Nourishing this newly acquired relationship with myself, worshiping it as the most important relationship, and myself, the most attractive person I can be with. I was called to meditate more, spend more time in silence.

I also stopped drinking. Suddenly alcohol seemed like toxic, useless chemicals floating in liquid. (This lasted for a few months and after that I went back to drinking very little.)

MY PATH: I believe in the power of psychedelic experiences so much that I plan to dedicate my career to it (by becoming a psychedelic integration coach and later, hopefully, a psychedelic therapist). I believe the versions of ourselves during psychedelics are more sober, awake, present, real, than the ones not on them.

In fact, during a past MDMA experience, I understood it like this: the Normal, "sober" of us are behind a door that is about 90% closed and only slightly open. And when we take psychedelics, the door opens and we can finally see what is always already there.

On psychedelics, we can understand, feel, and come to meet ourselves and others, for what we really are. We can see what is. Things that are always available to us though we cannot see through the blindfolds of beliefs, fears, noise, distractions, inhibitions...

In the future, I hope to work closer with Indigenous populations of South America and plant medicines. I aspire to become the vessel that bridges their ways to the West, a way to combine the two worlds through psychedelics. I truly genuinely want to work with them, learn from them, be around them.

I am now married... and you could say that Ayahuasca brought us together. He ended up coming with me to the ceremony, just for 2 out of 4 days, and I kept showing up in his visions. When the Taitas did the first healing and we sat next to each other, in his head, the Taita was marrying us in a way. After that, we became really good fiends – which eventually led to marriage.

Finally, from recent a MDMA experience and from microdosing: My mantra has become to simply appreciate beauty. The beauty of nature, of human civilization, of humans, of ourselves and life as a whole. And there does not need to be a purpose higher than that. To appreciate this life while we're passing by is enough. To be grateful. And present and hence alive.

FINAL THOUGHTS: Spending time with loved ones should be such an important priority for us, but life often gets in the way. Why does it take us our entire lives – or even taking psychedelics – to realize this lesson? We need to really focus on spending more quality time with those people who make our lives worth living – while we still have time.

EDITOR'S NOTES:

KEY TAKEAWAYS FROM ALEXANDRA'S STORY

- Most people seem to benefit from multiple ceremonies with Ayahuasca, as the medicine stays within the system for several days.
- Developing clear intentions – ones that become a mantra during challenging moments – is one of the most important things to accomplish prior to a ceremony.
- While the Indigenous traditions do not involve much integration, because of the ways of our Western cultures, we need to take the time to develop a framework for taking our revelations and insights and incorporating them into our everyday lives.
- Setting matters. For the truest experience with this medicine and the powerful healers/shamen who facilitate these ceremonies, people should travel to centers in South America, Mexico, or Costa Rica… plus, it's legal there.
- Psychedelic medicines help you to tap into parts of your brain and perceptions that are typically hidden/unavailable in normal consciousness.

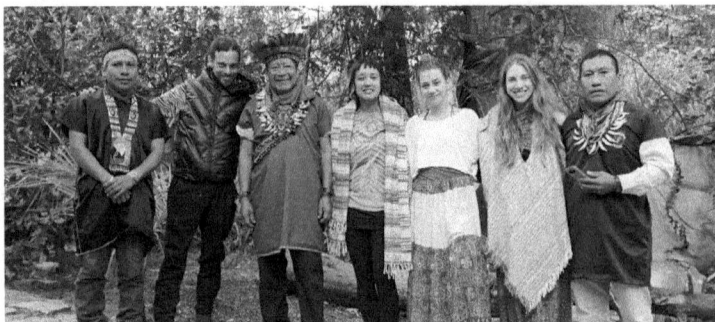

A photo of Alexandra (second, from right) and others at her retreat.

CHAPTER SEVENTEEN

Healing Story #14
I Sensed the Holy Spirit Moving Through My Body

STORYTELLER: Hunt, Male, White/Caucasian, Episcopal Priest, Gen X

MEDICINE CONSUMED: Psilocybin

DOSAGE: 3.5 grams

FOCUS/GOAL/INTENTION: To be open to what comes

BEST PART OF THIS JOURNEY: The embodied nature of the whole experience; an experience of God in my entire body, from the tips of my toes to the top of my head.

BIGGEST CHALLENGE OF JOURNEY: Being stuck in loops of worrying about people whom I hadn't talked to in a long time. It kept me from moving on in the experience. I finally had to "set them aside," promising myself I would come back to them the next day.

....

PROFOUND HEALING JOURNEY STORY DETAILS

In early 2016, I found myself lying on a sofa in Baltimore, forever changed. Over the course of the previous 6 hours and again a month later, I had a series of primary religious experiences that altered the course of my personal and professional life.

Occasioned by medium-high doses of pharmaceutical-grade psilocybin, the active ingredient in "magic mushrooms," these mystical experiences opened my eyes to an almost completely hidden wholeness in the world; a wholeness that I now know exists within me and all of creation.

As an Episcopal priest, I was a participant in the Johns Hopkins Religious Leaders Study, under the care of a team of people who were both passionate researchers and compassionate guides. During two 8-hour session days and in the integration work that followed, I came to know and experience God, the Universe, friends, family, and my own life in new and expansive ways.

Among the primary religious experiences (also referred to as mystical experiences or non-ordinary states of consciousness) occasioned by the entheogens: I spoke in tongues, sensed the Holy Spirit moving through my body, had my ordination to the priesthood completed, and found myself healed from what I now believe was chronic anxiety.

At various times in the sessions, I also experienced a reentering of events from my past. In one of these experiences, a painful childhood memory was healed when I revisited a 1975 family gathering and truly saw and came to know more fully my then middle-aged father and uncles through my now middle-aged eyes. What caused the shift, I think, is that in that session vignette, I looked around the room and realized how broken my father and my one uncle already were, and thought that all these years, I'd missed the bigger story of that weekend: All those adults were middle-aged – and the men were already trapped by alcoholism and unlived dreams, and by extension so too was my mother and one of my aunts.

Reflecting on these vignettes, I couldn't help but remember how Paul talks of love in 1 Corinthians 13:8-13: *Love never fails; but if there are gifts of prophecy, they will be done away with; if there are tongues, they will cease; if there is knowledge, it will be done away with. ⁹ For we know in part and prophesy in part; ¹⁰ but when the perfect comes, the partial will be done away with. ¹¹ When I was a child, I used to speak like a child, think like a child, reason like a child; when I became a man, I did away with childish things. ¹² For now we see in a mirror dimly, but then face to face; now I know in part, but then I will know fully, just as I also have been fully known. ¹³ But now faith, hope, and love remain, these three; but the greatest of these is love.*

At the beginning of my first session at Hopkins, things began slowly, with faint geometric shapes (triangles and squares) coming into view. I felt like I was ascending into streams and strands of light. As if some embracing force was pulling me upward and higher and faster, I went the more light and the more brilliant the colors. There were times when the light seemed like optic fibers. Other times like streamers or trails of light. The colors were mostly purple, green, blue. They were often brilliant and shimmering and at times they seemed like "electric" versions of the color. Distorted almost, or maybe charged with energy and exaggerated; saturated.

KEY INSIGHTS: I remember smiling a lot during this part of the session and from time to time laughing. I felt like I was surrounded by goodness. Several times I realized I had lost my sense of playfulness and that I have forgotten the importance of play. I resolved, at one point, to play more.

I was having trouble getting comfortable. My legs were driving me crazy and my face and ears itched and I just felt unusually twitchy. It sounds worse than it was, but I was uncomfortable. I focused on my breath and began rubbing my hands along the back of the couch—I liked how the material felt.

During that time, the music switched to intense drumming; I remember drumming along with it on my legs and stomach. And I began to feel the beat in my body. At some point, I felt a slight electric pulse in my right leg. I remembered it being the same spot I'd experienced the same sensation near the end of a Vipassana meditation retreat in late summer 2014.

Midway through that first session, I began to experience a sensation of something lodged inside me. Not understanding what it was, I imagined it to be energy that had to be released, but with no easy way out. The current of energy, subtle at first, formed in my pelvis and intensified as it moved up my spinal column. When it eventually became lodged near my larynx, a blockage was created which then expanded and began to feel impenetrable. The pressure was so intense that at one point I thought the skin around my Adam's apple was going to blow open.

In my mind, I struggled to break it up and quite unexpectedly (and uncharacteristically) began to speak in tongues, the spiritual gift mentioned by Paul in 1 Corinthians 14:1-25. It's not something I ever imagined myself doing.

Not long after, my physical discomfort caused me to become agitated, causing my guides to sense that I was struggling with something difficult. I told them something was trying to get out of me. After asking permission, one of the facilitators, Bill, placed his hands on the top of my head as I sometimes do when offering healing prayers and anointing a parishioner (the sacrament of Unction); the other facilitator, Darrick, sat at my feet and allowed me to press my legs against him as I had done for my wife when she was in labor with our son.

The blockage didn't fully clear, but as the psilocybin began to wear off, I knew that the blocked energy had mostly moved through me. In our conversation afterward I asked them what all that energy was about. Bill smiled and said, "In Christian language, I think we call that the Holy Spirit."

Later, I remembered Romans 8:22-24, which speaks of the first fruits of the Spirit and of the labor pains as "we wait for adoption, the redemption of our bodies."

The ritual act of laying on of hands is mentioned multiple times in both the Hebrew and Christian scriptures. (See Numbers 27:15–23, Deuteronomy 34:9, Acts 8:14–19, Acts 6:5–6,) For Christians, the laying on of hands is used sacramentally as part of healing rituals, Confirmations and ordinations. The connection to healing was pretty obvious for me, but the connection to the sacrament of Ordination was a recent epiphany.

The entire last part of the session felt like a combination of electrical charge, orgasm, thrashing, and gyrating – constriction and contraction – like I was being electrocuted, but not to the point of danger or real pain. It felt like something was being expelled or sent out from inside of me. Or that something needed to be expressed and the only way that could happen was through this intense process.

The entire session felt holy and throughout I sensed the presence of the Divine beyond what words or usual theological or spiritual language can describe. I didn't, and still don't, feel a strong need to try to put that part of it in words. It's as if I just assumed God was present in it, like I do in most situations – whether joyful or sad, painful or blissful. I felt enveloped by a sense of adventure, safety, confidence, love, peace, and joy. The Holy was part of it all.

This second session followed the same general pattern as the first: I saw and felt myself ascending into color, I spent a significant amount of time with important people in my life, both from my past and current relationships, and then my body became electrified and I experienced a long period of shaking, contractions and periods of screaming, chanting, and rocking my body.

I also found myself moving through rivulets of color, like ripples on the water. They were purple, blue and green and I felt like I was swimming through them. I marveled at their beauty as I moved through them. Then I found myself, my wife and son and extended family and maybe even friends, on a speed boat laughing and smiling as we zipped around a lake, jumping over waves and making large circles and figure 8s with the boat. I remember noticing that although the boat was smallish, it was full of everyone I loved.

Somehow, during the second session, I found myself on the sofa, moving back and forth between lying on my stomach and being in a kneeling position. I came to know, during the movement, that I was kneeling and then prostrating myself in front of the Universe. If a sacrament is "an outward sign of an inward and spiritual grace," then my call to leadership in the Christian community was affirmed and deepened.

There were two refrains that I heard multiple times during the second and third parts of the session. One was a mostly remembered line from a Mary Oliver poem called The Summer Day. The line is "Tell me, what is it you plan to do with your one wild and precious life." In my memory, the question was what are you going to do with your wild and wonderful life? The other line was from a song by Iris Dement that I first heard as part of the opening credits of an HBO series that my wife and I got hooked on this past fall called *The Leftovers*. The line I kept hearing from that was "Let the mystery be."

The grace-filled gift I received at Hopkins brought me spiritual growth, clarity about my vocation, emotional healing, and a desire to make the experience available to all who need and desire it.

Throughout the entire experience with this study, I felt comfortable, well-cared for, and peaceful.

PERSONAL BACKGROUND

Ordained to the priesthood in The Episcopal Church in 2005, I have served congregations in Atlanta, Seattle, and Savannah. Over the years I have been with hundreds of people in crisis and since my participation in the study, I have wished time and again for a way to offer an experience of psilocybin to people dealing with debilitating depression, traumatic stress, end of life distress or addiction.

I now feel called to commit myself to the work of helping to make these healing substances understood, trusted, accessible, and widely available.

My primary areas of interest at the intersection of Christianity, current scientific research, and the Psychedelic Renaissance are:

using new and existing ritual and sacramental theology as well as fresh exegesis of sacred texts to empower Christians and other religious people to facilitate and expand the transformation that is possible with entheogens

incorporating entheogens as a trusted modality used by laypeople and clergy in their own healing and the healing of others

gathering a Christian community that encourages and values mystical experiences, including but not limited to those occasioned by entheogens.

POWERFUL INSIGHT: We in the West have been in a spiritual and emotional crisis for such a long time that our depression, addiction, and anxiety are nearly normalized. The trauma of the past year has only exacerbated what was already an epidemic of despair. Unfortunately, our current medical, psychological, and spiritual resources are not enough to heal and transform us.

I am hopeful that through education and acceptance of the transformative power of non-ordinary states of consciousness, Christians will embrace the possibilities that entheogens hold for spiritual growth and physical and mental health. Healing the sick and the transformation of all people was at the core of Jesus' earthly ministry. It must be at the core of ours as well.

EDITOR'S NOTES:

KEY TAKEAWAYS FROM HUNT'S STORY

- While, at the time of publication, all psychedelics are illegal at the federal level, there are legal clinical trials and scientific studies being conducted with these psychedelic medicines.

- Psychedelic journeys often lead to revisiting childhood traumas – but seeing them through a completely different lens, which leads to great healing and understanding.

- Depending on the dosage, many people experience profound spiritual/mystical healing and experiences when intentionally consuming these psychedelic medicines.

- With psychedelic medicines, journeyers often return with a new perspective on friends, family – and themselves.

- One of several mental health conditions that these psychedelic medicines help heal is chronic anxiety.

OTHER DETAILS

Hunt Priest is Episcopal priest working at the intersection of contemplative Christianity and sacred plants and fungi. He is Executive Director and Founder of Ligare, an open network of people who desire legal and safe access and believe that Christianity and other existing religious traditions offer paths for preparing, experiencing, and integrating mystical experiences, including those occasioned by sacred plants and compounds. URL: https://www.ligare.org/

The Summer Day

Who made the world?
Who made the swan, and the black bear?
Who made the grasshopper?
This grasshopper, I mean
the one who has flung herself out of the grass,
the one who is eating sugar out of my hand,
who is moving her jaws back and forth instead of up and down
who is gazing around with her enormous and complicated eyes.
Now she lifts her pale forearms and thoroughly washes her face.
Now she snaps her wings open, and floats away.
I don't know exactly what a prayer is.
I do know how to pay attention, how to fall down
into the grass, how to kneel down in the grass,
how to be idle and blessed, how to stroll through the fields,
which is what I have been doing all day.
Tell me, what else should I have done?
Doesn't everything die at last, and too soon?
Tell me, what is it you plan to do
with your one wild and precious life?

—MARY OLIVER

Let the Mystery Be

Everybody's wonderin' what and where
They all came from
Everybody's worryin' 'bout where they're gonna go
When the whole thing's done
But no one knows for certain and so it's all the same to me
I think I'll just let the mystery be
Some say once gone you're gone forever
And some say you're gonna come back
Some say you rest in the arms of the Savior
If in sinful ways you lack
Some say that they're comin' back in a garden
Bunch of carrots and little sweet peas
I think I'll just let the mystery be
Everybody's wonderin' what and where
They all came from
Everybody's worryin' 'bout where they're gonna go
When the whole thing's done
But no one knows for certain and so it's all the same to me
I think I'll just let the mystery be
Some say they're goin' to a place called Glory
And I ain't saying it ain't a fact
But I've heard that I'm on the road to Purgatory
And I don't like the sound of that
I believe in love and I live my life accordingly
But I choose to let the mystery be

–IRIS DEMENT

CHAPTER EIGHTEEN

Healing Story #15
Coming Out of the Psychedelic Closet, or...
Diving in Deep Into The Unknown

STORYTELLER: Bea, Female, BIPOC/Chinese, Entrepreneur, Millennial

MEDICINE CONSUMED: Ayahuasca/DMT

DOSAGE: 1 cup

FOCUS/GOAL/INTENTION: After discussing with trusted friends, here were my intentions:

- Think of what you intentionally want to bring into your life and one thing you want to let go of
- Show me who I've become (not how I see myself or others do, but who I am)
- Merge me back with my soul at all costs
- Heal my heart

BEST PART OF THIS JOURNEY: Self-love, encouragement, downloads

BIGGEST CHALLENGE OF JOURNEY: Fear, anxiety, self-doubt, dying

....

PROFOUND HEALING JOURNEY STORY DETAILS

Around my late 20s, I found myself in a career I didn't enjoy anymore – I had material success but not fulfillment – and I was experiencing the loss of my grandpa, whom I was very close to.

So I did the most logical thing... in 2018, I bought a one-way ticket to Asia, to my ancestral lands. I lived and worked in Hong Kong, Macau, China, Japan, Taiwan, and Thailand while embarking on a path of self-discovery.

Luckily, I fell into a group of friends who were spiritually-curious and I ended up learning a lot from them about self-care, mindset, and establishing a good morning and evening ritual. Somewhere along the way, I was introduced to psychedelics.

My first time was in Pai, Thailand, where I drank a mushroom shake; but I didn't get the experience everybody was telling me about… so, I tried a second time. The next time, I bought some dried mushrooms about the size of my palm in Koh Phangan. All I felt was maybe a slight buzz and nothing more.

So I thought maybe psychedelics weren't meant for me and I moved on.

Fast forward a few years later, at the height of the pandemic (circa summer 2020), I came back home to Canada – only to realize I wasn't ready to be back yet… so I went down to Mexico, the only open country at the time.

I once again fell into a group of spiritually-forward people who were pro-psychedelic and taught me all about set and setting, dosage, safety, and intentions.

Diving deep into plant medicines, I participated in my first 5-MeO-DMT ceremony, followed by an Ayahuasca journey just two weeks later.

I did the 5-MeO-DMT [one of the most intense psychedelic experiences] before Ayahuasca… because I was scared of Aya. The feedback from my friends about Aya was mixed; half said it's the best thing ever and the other half told me their horror stories.

The 5-MeO was indeed powerful. After taking the medicine, I immediately collapsed onto my mat and became one with the Earth… while I argued with myself in my head if I was doing the journey "right" – and actually experienced ego death. I took away many lessons from that journey alone!

After the 5-MeO ceremony, I felt as ready as I possibly could be for Aya. I still had some concerns – like what if some suppressed childhood memory came up and I wasn't ready to deal with it? Or what if I have a psychotic breakdown? I mean, do I really want to open Pandora's Box?

I moved forward with an overnight stay in the jungle in Mexico. I signed up for this particular ceremony because the facilitator was a trained musician who had toured the world before he shifted to plant medicine work. It was quite a treat as all night long so many beautiful healing Icaros were played.

EDITOR'S NOTE: Icaro means "song," or more specifically, a sacred medicine song. Icaros are specific to certain regions and teachers/healers, and are sung in different languages. Icaros are seen as powerful tools that help with healing, calling on the healing properties of the plants.

For preparation, I took the dieta seriously for about a week and fasted 24 hours before.

At the ceremony, we began with a four-directions prayer – sending our gratitude to the east, west, north and south, to Father Sky and Mother Earth – then we were served Rapé (a powerful, cleansing snuff used by shamans). Consuming anything by nose is very uncomfortable for me, but the shaman promised it would be the most gentle experience I'd ever have – and he was right.

Then, one by one, we drank a cup of Ayahuasca. When I finished drinking and sat back down, people before me were already purging.

By the way, it tasted horrible. It was sour, bitter, gritty with dirt. Definitely not my favorite drink!

There was an open fire burning beside us that gave us light and warmth. I laid down on my yoga mat and looked up to the sky, past the trees – the sun was setting and the moon was getting ready to shine.

The beginning of my journey was a bit scary. In my mind's eye, my body was completely paralyzed on the ground. All of a sudden, all these creepy crawlies – bugs like cockroaches, ants, and spiders (ugh, gross!) – came out of nowhere and started eating my body alive. I tried to get up, but couldn't move. I tried to shout for help, but couldn't speak. There was nothing I could do about it… I couldn't save myself and my life depended on it.

So, I decided to just surrender and welcome my imminent death.

And the minute I stopped struggling and accepted reality, that's when my journey did a 180 and I shot up into bliss.

Instead of throwing up like other participants, my way of purging was through yawning.

Yawn after yawn after yawn. Each yawn produced a galaxy into the universe – whole solar systems were coming out of my being! The message here was: I am the creator of my life, so I'm in charge of my reality (we all are!). If I don't like it, I have full control to change it." It felt empowering to know that.

Sometime later, I entered another dimension; I don't even know how to describe it.

When my eyes were open, the moon turned into my grandma. It was as if I reverted back into a baby and was looking up at my grandma from my crib. She was cooing at me – her adorable grandbaby – and it felt so loving.

I saw all this through these beautiful, translucent patterns with a rainbow sheen – similar to the surface of a soap bubble. A friend of mine later told me they were called the *Shipibo Knots* – I have yet to confirm that through my own research.

When I closed my eyes, I didn't see much visuals but instead received downloads of information.

For example, I had a deep knowing that I've been Asian in many, many past lives – that's why I'm so comfortable and proud of being Chinese in my current life. In my past lives, I've been an empress, a wealthy merchant, and a member of the royal family, etc.

The message to me here was: *success is in your cards, so why are you doubting yourself?*

Throughout the night, these waves of self-love were pouring out of me and going back into myself. I saw an older, wiser version of myself who kept shaking her head at me and playfully say "silly girl, you're so silly (to doubt yourself)."

At one point during the ceremony, two women I didn't know had somehow rolled over into my space. Their limbs were touching me – one of them even used me as her pillow. I was going to say something but then I realized both of them were crying. They were at a low point in their journey – releasing whatever they didn't need to carry anymore – while I was at a high point. So, I decided to allow it to happen. If my small discomfort can bring them some relief in their time of need, why not? It's the least that I can do.

I had the opportunity to go up for a second dose, which I considered as I had come down a bit, but decided not to. It felt like I had one foot firmly planted back in reality while the other was still in la-la-land… and I didn't feel the need or desire to completely untether from reality.

At the end of the ceremony, we all gathered around the open fire – drinking water, eating fruit, and humming along to the beautiful music.

I had a wondrous time feeling an immense amount of love from my higher self, laughing innocently like a little kid, and exploring the depths of my fears, my truths, and my mind.

My Ayahuasca journey was nothing short of magical. In fact, it was the genesis of me coming out of the psychedelic closet and jumping with both feet into the industry. About 7 months later, I co-founded Sisters in Psychedelics (SIP), a social enterprise with a mission to empower people to elevate the divine feminine and other underrepresented voices in the evolution of the psychedelic ecosystem.

A note on integration here. I think North Americans (myself included) tend to overcomplicate things. From what I was told, the Indigenous people's integration protocol is simply to consistently be in community. So, how I facilitated integration for myself has mostly been: journaling and telling my friends about my psychedelic experiences, my downloads, and my lessons learned. Those "aha" moments are so important to remember! Then, I reflect on what I can incorporate into my life on a regular basis that will help me unlock the next level in this game of life. Finally, I take action and do it.

PERSONAL BACKGROUND

I had a pretty typical Asian upbringing – you know, my childhood was very structured, very strict. It was an environment where everything you do or say was scrutinized and you're regularly told you're not good enough –that really had a big impact on my self-worth, self-esteem.

There was also domestic violence and emotional neglect within the family, and all the things that come with being an immigrant family; for example, being seen as different and experiencing racism from others, sexism from within my own culture, pressure from parents to succeed even at the expense of myself, cultural and generational gap from within the home, learning English and Chinese at the same time, and trying to fit into the Western society with Eastern views and values influenced from home.

Lastly, there's societal brainwashing to fit the mold… go to university, get a good job, buy that house, get married, have kids, do this, do that.

On the flip side, I was very lucky to grow up with 3 of my 4 grandparents up until my mid-20s. I was much closer to my maternal grandparents, so when my grandpa passed, that sparked me to quit my job and spend time in Asia. His death was the first death I experienced in life – it was a wake-up, because if he could die, then so could my parents – and so could I… so, why am I spending time doing things I don't enjoy?

Psychedelics have also helped me with ancestral healing. For example, my mom's mom, my grandmother, tells stories of running away from the Japanese invasion of China when she was only four. And my grandpa? He was put in jail by Chairman Mao during the cultural revolution in communist China – just for being a teacher.

So my mother grew up without her father while my grandma became a single working mom raising three kids on her own. Furthermore, when my mother was 15, she was ripped away from her family and thrown to the countryside for years to do agricultural work as part of Mao's re-education through manual labor regime.

It was all very traumatizing to that entire generation in China! No doubt the psychological and emotional impact lingered and has been passed down to the next generation (Millennials, like me).

One particular LSD journey really helped me understand, forgive, and accept my mom as who she is. We're a lot closer now as a result of developing empathy and compassion for her.

My hope is that by being vulnerable and sharing my personal story, it can help other people in their path of healing, no matter what healing modality they use.

KEY THOUGHT: YOUR UPBRINGING IS NOT YOUR DESTINY.

One very interesting aside in the discussion of psychedelics in the Asian language – and I'm talking about Chinese, Korean, Japanese etc. – is that most psychedelic terms do not exist. And for the very few that do, they have negative connotations to it. For example, the word psychedelics is 迷幻藥, which translates to "hallucinogenic meditation," but which really means "illegal narcotics." And MDMA? It's 搖頭丸 which translates into "shaking head pill" because young people use it at raves. I mean, how do you even talk about psychedelics with your family if the words don't even exist?

I think it's time for a rebrand and one of the pet projects I'm working on would be to (re)create more accurate terms in Chinese. If anyone is interested in collaborating with me on this, please connect with me at bea@sistersinpsychedelics. org. I'd be happy to hear from you!

FINAL WORDS OF ADVICE: Do your research. Conduct internet searches, watch YouTube videos, listen to podcasts. Get your hands on as much content from different sources as you can. Talk to people – your friends, friends of friends. You could even do what I did – put out a post on social media asking for advice… crowdsourcing at its finest!

Also, locate and join your local psychedelic society; many cities have them, but if yours doesn't, then find an online community. This is one reason we created Sister in Psychedelics – a place for community, engagement, sharing, and asking questions. *Community is essential.*

Remember too, that your first step into psychedelics might be microdosing – getting to know the medicine first before going on a full journey with a macrodose. With microdosing, you really don't feel any kind of impact beyond being more open, more productive; you're completely functional, which is why people microdosed on LSD in Silicon Valley for years.

EDITOR'S NOTES:

KEY TAKEAWAYS FROM BEA'S STORY

- Regardless of which method you plan to use to consume one of these psychedelic medicines – in a clinical trial, in a healing center, with a coach, or by yourself – it is truly essential to complete your due diligence of finding all the necessary research before jumping into the medicine.

- Whether we realize it or not, we all carry the trauma from our parents, grandparents, and so on; it's called generational trauma (but also known as intergenerational trauma or transgenerational trauma). For immigrant families, that trauma can become stifling, overwhelming.

- While all these psychedelic medicines have similar properties and pathways to healing and understanding, you may have to try more than one to obtain the healing/answers you seek.

- These medicines are not only beneficial for healing, but many people – typically on higher doses – gain brilliant insights and ideas from their journeys… something we refer to as digital downloads.

OTHER DETAILS

Bea Chan is the co-founder of Sisters In Psychedelics (SIP), a grassroots-to-global social enterprise birthed in Vancouver, Canada, to create a more balanced, inclusive and accessible psychedelic ecosystem for today and for generations to come. "Our offerings are primarily for women and we welcome all genders too." Join our community here: www.sistersinpsychedelics.org

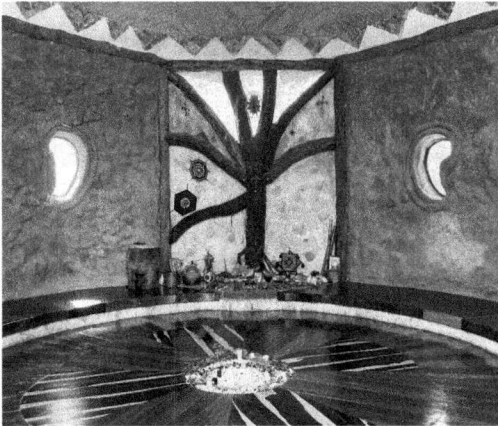

A photo of Bea's ceremonial space.

CHAPTER NINETEEN

Healing Story #16
My Ego Witnessed Itself for What it Was:
Clever, Deceitful, and Powerful

STORYTELLER: Tuscany, Female, White/Caucasian, Millennial

MEDICINE CONSUMED: Psilocybin

DOSAGE: 3.5 g, 1 tbsp. in powder form, with cocoa

FOCUS/GOAL/INTENTION: to have my eyes open and see interconnectivity or mingling of energy

BEST PART OF THIS JOURNEY: the insight that my ego is tricking me most of the time

BIGGEST CHALLENGE OF JOURNEY: the insight that my ego is tricking me most of the time

....

PROFOUND HEALING JOURNEY STORY DETAILS

I was nervous around psychedelics up until about a year ago because I had a couple of psychedelic experiences where I felt I didn't quite have control, physically and mentally. The medicine felt pushed on me a little bit, like, "You'll like it. It's not a big deal. You don't need all day" – with little detail offered around what I was getting into. Also, I would usually get a headache or stomachache as the medicine was being digested as well as during and after a journey.

These experiences were never bad, but I carried with me the importance of having enough time to reintegrate, to be in the right setting and to know more about the dosage I was taking. I never researched psychedelics extensively before any of my journeys. Looking back this seems silly. I suppose I was just "doing the research" by my own experimentation. I had done some quick online searches but overall, I got most of my information from word-of-mouth.

For this particular journey, I was with two friends, one very close to me and experienced with psilocybin and one somewhat close to me and not very experienced (she was taking less, about 1 gram).

Both people I felt I could be vulnerable with. Very important to me. I also cleared my schedule and was out of my home environment in a cozy cabin that felt safe. Also very important to me because I have a teenage child, and so I always want to eliminate as many possible emergencies as I can.

I had been sourcing from the same person for about a year by now. The medicine was shipped from California, some in gummy form or capsules for microdosing and some in pouches. The pouches included 7 grams of ground psilocybin mixed with cocoa (apparently cocoa helps with activating the medicine sooner). For this journey, I mixed a tablespoon, half of the pouch, with a small glass of kombucha and drank it in about 5-10 minutes.

I had done this type of medicine enough times by now, that for this particular journey I didn't feel the need to worry about certain music or lighting. I just needed chill people (which I had, yes!). We gave each other space and also checked in on each other. I spent most of my time in a lawn chair on the porch or inside in a recliner.

I started by sitting on the porch and let the medicine flow through me. I watched the breeze through the trees and breathed while I adjusted. It usually takes me 30-45 minutes to adjust. During this time it seems most beneficial to be super comfortable, usually sitting, and not talking to anyone. I started to see the trees blend and play with my mind. Although that was fun to observe, I love observing my body sensations too, especially when I have pain of any sort. I currently had neck pain, which was common for me. I went into it.

I closed my eyes and just felt it. I played here for a while. I could move it, intensify it or let it float away. I also drifted in and out of listening to the birds and sounds around me. I felt like they engulfed me – or we were one of the same? Were my arms my arms? Where were my arms? Was that sound in me or out of me? I suppose that was a form of wholeness? I don't know! I was definitely one with sound. But I just couldn't get myself to open my eyes and maintain focus to explore that experience more. I moved into the living room.

My mindset was fairly stable and open, although a conversation the previous day had perplexed me, and made me overly motivated to understand wholeness. The conversation was about the actions of enlightened people and how being enlightened means you have a certain sensitivity to the world. The premise was, if you're enlightened, then you understand your connection to all things, therefore there is a sensitivity in you and you don't want to hurt other living things.

I felt like I understood that, but then are all these enlightened people frauds? Don't we all have blind spots? What does "connection to all things" really look like? Why do I always hear about people seeing energy and knowing that we're all connected? Why had I heard about people having experiences, with their eyes open, where they observed objects, their external world, blending together?

Had I even experienced wholeness? Did I even know what this label meant? These were the questions floating in my thoughts during my journey.

I didn't just want to understand wholeness through thought, I wanted to "see" it. I wanted to see wholeness as a truth, not just a trip mind trick where the floor is moving and shapes are blending, but as true reality. I thought that if I saw this, I would possibly understand what people meant by wholeness and energy. Don't get me wrong, I had some other crazy experiences on psychedelics in which I felt egoless and "okay with all things", but I was looking for something different.

I thought that with my eyes open I could practice, and really feel, how to live in that place of wholeness, not just get a glimpse. I felt like I needed one of these "unity experiences" to understand spirituality and what it's all about. The funny thing is, I never defined myself as a spiritual seeker; I just wanted to know Truth. But here I was, seeking. I felt like I was on the verge of understanding... something.

I decided I wanted to be quiet. I started to drift into a quiet place and back to my questions: Are we really all connected? What is all this wholeness stuff about? My mind was focused and open.

Then, it started. My mind started checking off my ego's tricks in a conclusive sort of way... My desire to "be a good person"? Trick. My fear of death? Trick. The idea OF death? Trick. Spiritual culture? Bullshit! Anxiety? Fear = Trick. Most of my thoughts are useful and needed? Lie. Trick. I AM my thoughts? Trick. I'm pretty far on this so-called enlightenment journey? Not even close. The things I do that I label as "meaningful" are meaningful? Trick. The things other people label as "meaningful" are meaningful? Trick. The problems humans face are separate? Nope. I know how to help the world's problems and I am helping!? Trick.

It was insane. It was like a hurricane filled with droplets of my ego's lies. Ego isn't only evident when we think things like, "Oh, my hair is ugly. I wish my hair looked like that," it's also evident when I think, "I deserve more than that ant," or "I should advocate for peace" or "I'm scared of death." Who says you're more important than that ant? Who says you should care about world peace? Why would you be scared of death if not for your ego? Yes, your ego dies (and it really doesn't want to!), but do *you?* What is *you?* Could death be nothing more than a transition? Well, ego will tell you otherwise, that's for sure.

I started to cry as the lies slammed down on me and buried me in overwhelming sadness and grief. I could open my eyes at this point. I could look around and see that it didn't matter if my eyes were open or closed. It didn't matter if I "saw" wholeness or had some radical spiritual experience. Those were just my ego's tricks, too!

I cried in disbelief for about twenty minutes as I breathed in the realization: Ego and Maya's power reigns over all of us. All my beliefs are wrong. All a joke. All the things I worry about and think about are silly. Super silly! I know what it means to wake up, to be enlightened, and I am not. There is an end to this game; there is true seeing. I'm just beginning and all I thought I knew was nothing special. The hurricane was subsiding and a clarity remained: My ego has been tricking me this whole time.

EDITOR'S NOTE: Spiritual traditions of India commonly teach that the world is Maya – translated as 'illusion' or 'unreality.' That the world is Maya is the basis of the emphasis on yoga and meditation in Indian thought, which is regarded as the means of moving beyond Maya

There is further to go and there is an end. Ego tricks us easily here; it says one of two things: 1) "Yup, life is a journey, man, there is no end." False. This is ego trying to get us to ignore truth and stay in our comfort zones. 2) "I'm there! I'm awake!" False. Unless you are. And the bus-like experience taught me that very few people are awake. Very, very few. Like, maybe 500 people. Jed McKenna (a pseudonym for an author of a series of books on enlightenment) says maybe 20 or so. I choose a higher estimate, either way, now that I know ego and Maya's power, I know it is very hard to attain and much easier to be tricked into thinking we attained it.

The psilocybin helped me get the first glimpse of what true spirituality means.

What really stinks is that now I realize I know something; I also realize I know practically nothing. I have so much further to go! The journey really just began.

After the journey, I was able to receive hugs and comfort after my insight. I was also in the cabin for another day so I was able to go for walks and wonder out loud with my friends. One outstanding learning from this journey is that I don't need to remember anything anymore, just quiet time seems essential.

I also happened to pick up a book that was describing exactly what I was going through, Jed McKenna's *Spiritual Enlightenment: The Damndest Thing.* This helped me understand my experience and remember to keep going. There is no more a need to plan action or do anything (oh the paradoxes!).

I saw the truth about the ego so clearly that all effort *is* the ego. This is the trap. All I can do is continue to pause on thoughts and actions, and question their reality and need. I must slow down and figure this spirituality stuff out on my own. I now know the answer is simple and not in thought but in a quiet place that has always been with me, but my thoughts battle daily now with this puzzle. The integration will continue until I've arrived or given up.

MY ADVICE: Set and setting: know what you're taking and don't get stuck on your intention. Flow, adjust and breathe. You can go deep into the psyche and it's complex in there. Changing your setting or having a trusted support to help you reframe the challenging moment is necessary sometimes.

PERSONAL BACKGROUND

I have a partner whose life has been positively affected greatly from psychedelics. He has helped me see the benefits of the medicine and how it can have life-altering effects. Psychedelics have changed my life – helped me overcome headaches and sleepwalking related to anxiety.

We both see psychedelics as a truth-realizing medicine. We take it solely for this reason: to observe what is true vs not true.

I can honestly say that psychedelics are a part of my life. When the timing works out, I partake.

About a year ago, I planned and prepped the heck out of my psyche and environment and did a large dose of psilocybin, about 7 grams, with a trusted partner as my support. The experience was insightful and beautiful, although I did struggle with one of the worst headaches of my life, and body aches and weakness, during the journey and the next day.

I've done one other 7-gram dose and two 3.5-gram doses since then. I now understand my body and the medicine better. To avoid stomachaches, body aches and headaches, I make sure to eat a healthy meal about a half-an-hour before I dose, and I drink a lot of water throughout and afterward, usually mixed with electrolytes, teas or green powders.

My time on psilocybin has been easier, less prep needed, less aches and less anxiety. I also find 3-3.5 grams is my sweet spot. I don't get headaches, stomachaches (although sometimes as the medicine is digesting, I feel slightly nauseous) and fewer body aches (although they are there), and the insights are just as profound.

In terms of other issues, I was never a spiritual seeker, but I was always curious. I was never into gems, chanting, the moon, astrology, tarot cards, or any new age ideas. I did one 10-day silent vipassana retreat to try to get rid of my headaches and I am certified in yoga in case I need a side job. I'm not sure I could have had this experience if my ego was attached to the spirituality industry. On the other hand, I'm not sure I could have had this experience if I knew nothing about certain spiritual concepts.

I also have experience meditating, doing yoga, and I had one psilocybin trip where I got the cosmic giggles and saw all the silliness in our reality. (I mentioned this journey earlier, 7 grams, about a year ago). I felt egoless and was okay with death.

EDITOR'S NOTES:

KEY TAKEAWAYS FROM TUSCANY'S STORY

- While set and setting are extremely important, if you experience yourself in a challenging situation, try changing one or both – breathe through the experience and consider changing locations to something more comfortable/safe.

- Diving inward can lead to insights, but it can feel scary. Having a trusted supportive person with you can make all the difference when feeling fear and anxiety, and to process the experience afterward.

- We all have a shadow (dark) self/side driven by our egos.

- On higher doses, many people taking psychedelic medicines experience spiritual occurrences/awakenings.

- Cacao has been consumed as a sacred drink for thousands of years for its heart-opening properties; it also contains MAO-inhibitors that increase and lengthen the effect of psilocybin, which is why some people mix the two. Cacao generally refers to the ground seeds of the Cacao fruit; it contains healthy fats that carry many essential nutrients. When the butter is removed from the Cacao, the solid powder left behind is known as "cocoa powder." This cocoa powder is used by the confectionery industry and in the making of cheap chocolate, usually by infusing it with lower quality vegetable fats.

CHAPTER TWENTY

Healing Story #17
I Could Not Compromise My Truth Any Longer

STORYTELLER: Katja, Female, White/Caucasian, Millennial

MEDICINE CONSUMED: Ayahuasca

DOSAGE: 1 serving (from Shaman) – (1 big dose)

FOCUS/GOAL/INTENTION: What does the medicine want/desire from me?

BEST PART OF THIS JOURNEY: The visuals and intense colors, as well as synesthesia

BIGGEST CHALLENGE OF JOURNEY: None

....

PROFOUND HEALING JOURNEY STORY DETAILS

This psychedelic experience was my first – ever. I never had any other touch-points with psychedelics or any other mind-altering substances except one cigarette and 3 puffs of weed as a teen – even though I had been living in Berlin for 12 years; Berlin has a big party scene.

I ended up staying a total of four days in the jungle with just one other person and the shaman and his helper. It was my initial encounter with plant medicine; the first time with Ayahuasca. I had no idea what Ayahuasca was at the time – the medicine found me. More interestingly, when I showed up, the shaman already knew that I was coming –- without knowing I was coming.

I was nervous. And somehow, I knew this experience was going to change my life… and I was ready to do it. So there was a lot of fear, and it took a leap of faith to actually do the first journey. I knew I felt ready – and I knew something was coming. But I also know now and sensed it back then: it's always good to approach the medicine with respect and humbleness. I see it as more than just a hedonistic psychedelic trip that is fun.

The first night of ceremony – and I don't even consider it my first journey – I purged right after consuming the medicine and that was the end of my night. All the pre-ceremonial tobacco tea I had to drink earlier (used for a tobacco cleanse before sacred ceremonies) had already made me a bit queasy even before consuming the medicine.

An interesting side note: I would say, looking back, that in two-thirds of the journeys, I don't even purge anymore. It's as though my body has developed a different way of purging – more like soft purging through yawning or shaking – but not the physical vomiting.

Ah, but the second night… on my first real journey, the world revealed itself to me – a world that I knew had always existed from childhood, but which had become a bit lost in adulthood.

I knew the journey was starting when it felt like something was dripping on my third eye inside. And then a big drop opened up the vision. For me, the way the medicine communicates with me is very visual.

My experience felt like coming back home; it was as if the spiritual world was welcoming me back – with fireworks. I had synesthesia (in which information meant to stimulate one of your senses stimulates several of your senses), and could see sounds as colors and perceive multidimensionality visually.

I had so many amazing, crazy visuals and the journey itself was super powerful. Amazingly, the shaman was with me in the journey so he could see what I was seeing. We later talked about it – and the ability to take so much time to talk about what I experienced really helped with integration… and I also had time to ask myself the big questions.

The journey was quite amazing – and really, I had no challenges. I believe I cried a few tears, as I often do on journeys, but nothing challenging.

That said, perhaps the takeaways from the journey were the most challenging. The end result from this experience was that I needed to change the direction of my life quite drastically.

One thing that became clear was that I had to leave my 12-year relationship – even though he's an amazing man – we had been together for more than a decade; I could have easily stayed with him the next 40 years just because we got along so well, but I could never develop into the person I was supposed to become by being at his side.

That was such a tough decision to make because it felt like choosing between the relationship and me and I knew it would be hurting him so deeply. I didn't even have a real reason or explanation that would satisfy the rational mind except that it felt like the right thing.

Another thing that came through for me from the medicine was I could not continue doing what I'm doing professionally; I had spent the previous years of my life in corporate marketing.

I needed to turn my career to something that has more purpose – something that is actually bringing more good into the world. (At the time I was working in fashion public relations for a big e-commerce retailer, doing all these fun projects, fashion weeks and parties, drinking champagne with the talent and influencers, but it was not really contributing to making the world a better place.)

I knew I had to do something in that direction, but didn't really know what that would look like. I didn't think of coaching back then, but I also knew I would need to integrate spirituality more into my work. I had no clue how, and was so afraid to do it because I'd been spiritual for a while, but never really had a coming out because I was too afraid of how people might judge me or what they might say.

Before the ceremony, I also had numerous fears, especially of spiders and things that crawl. And afterward, I was sitting on this stone at a waterfall, enjoying the beauty of nature, with the jungle behind me. Then it hit me – something feels different. I looked around and realized how calm I was. Previous to the medicine, I would have been afraid that a snake might bite me or something might crawl on me. That fear or phobia had somehow modified itself without me even setting an intention.

Another profound shift I noticed was how the medicine put me more in touch with my intuition. Afterward, my goal was really just to follow the intuitive signs, and those have guided me on my path forward.

Interesting side note: Back then, the shaman told me, "You're not new to this; I don't have to tell you. And whenever you want to go down that path and learn, I would be willing to teach you." I was stunned and excited – and thanked him for the offer.

Somehow, I knew that I would pick him up on this offer – but not until sometime later – which I then did!

After the ceremonies, I went home to make all those really difficult decisions. I ended that relationship. I decided on a career change not knowing what that new career would be… so it felt a bit like suicide of my old identity on so many levels – because it was not just one area of life; *It was a complete change on all levels.*

I just surrendered to that feeling of being lost and not knowing what the next steps look like and also allowing that – and being okay with that. Then, by coincidence, I came across this coaching school. I had never considered coaching as an option, but was drawn to it energetically and by my curiosity.

At the same time, I took another corporate job to basically buy myself time to transition out into what I wanted to do next. Obtaining the coaching degree and enjoying the work with people in this way a lot, I decided to transition into that field as my next step. After a year, I left that corporate job and decided to become self-employed – right at the time when the pandemic hit.

Luckily, around that same time, I heard that my shaman had moved to a place in Mexico that had been drawing me in for years – and I knew that now the time had come for me to learn. So I went there with the intention to do something he referred to as *a shamanic initiation/shamanic priestess* initiation for two months and work intensely with the medicine as well. Those two months turned into four months – living with him and his partner and really diving deeply into the medicine work with Aya, but also with other master plants.

During this time, I changed so much. I became more in touch with my feminine energy and came more into balance – really arriving at myself. I also knew the medicine would somehow be part of my future work, although I didn't see myself administering it; that was not my path.

So I decided to leave Germany and moved to Mexico and then things fell in place even further – and led to what I'm basically doing now, combining coaching and plant medicine. I'm a leadership coach with a degree in transformation coaching. I'm also a psychedelic preparation and integration guide and host 1:1 private and group retreats – which can, but don't have to, be plant medicine-assisted.

KEY INSIGHT: Instead of lifestyle experiences for brands, I now design and facilitate transformative experiences for humans who want to grow and find more meaning and connection.

It's kind of amazing, looking back. From the corporate world and really being rooted in one timeline and one completely different life to… now living in the jungle on a property where there's tranquility and the monkeys come by and visit during the day.

My life is so very different now, but I feel it's way more me and way more authentic and I owe the medicine so much. I'm so, so grateful for the path it put me on – even if it wasn't easy, and even if it meant doing all of the uncomfortable work.

PERSONAL BACKGROUND

I had a near-death experience when I was little; when I was in kindergarten. I almost drowned – and in that moment, I was literally seeing this movie of my life; all of the beautiful memories of everything and everyone that's been relevant passed in front of me like a movie. Then I experienced a sensation of being in a tunnel – where there's light at the end – and it felt quite warm and not really frightening.

Since that accident, I'm not really afraid of death. I'm afraid of pain but I'm not afraid of death or dying because I know that there's more – beyond death. And this got me really curious about what's beyond.

I was always exploring and reading and being curious, but more for myself. I also was lucky to meet the right people in my early twenties; I met a woman who was a kind of a healer, and she started an intuitive women's circle where she taught me how to train my heightened senses and tap into it. I also learned more about energetic protection – and how to protect myself and not let energies affect me if I don't want them to.

And the more I opened up to these things, the more the right people came into my life – as well as some interesting synchronicities and beautiful intuitive insights.

So that's been my spiritual journey. I would say I've always been spiritual; I could show you a picture of me as a like a kid in kindergarten, which I found last year – and if you look at my eyes, I look like I have the eyes of a 70-year-old woman. And the look I have is like… *guys you have no idea what you're getting yourself into.*

And I feel the older I get, also of course the more conscious I become, and the more I have worked with the medicine, the more my inner child comes out… and I approach life with play, with that sense of the inner child.

So… how did I end up in the jungle, participating in a ceremony in the Mexican jungle?

Well, it started when my company had a mass firing; while they didn't fire me, they did fire about half of my team – some of whom were close friends. I was so disappointed that I thought I would inquire about getting my own severance package; everybody was getting three months of salary and they were talking about using the time to travel.

I was supposed to get a promotion and pick up the broken pieces from the mass firing, but I didn't feel it at all. I went to HR and just wanted to inquire about the solution and I still don't know what happened, but two minutes later

I walked out – having signed my resignation letter. It was quite an intuitive impulse decision, but it felt good.

The next week, on my first morning off, I was lying in bed thinking about what I had done and worrying that I was never going to find a good job again. I was getting myself worked up so I decided I was too stressed out and needed to go on vacation and gather myself. I checked flights, found a really good flight to one of my favorite spots in Mexico, but I knew I didn't want to just lay on the beach in Tulum like always; I needed to see something different. I looked at the map and Palenque caught my eye; it's an archeological site in the jungle, about 10 hours away from where I was planning to stay.

I just knew something amazing, something very relevant, would happen when I visited there. Yes, I would do some sight-seeing and relax, but there was something more. Amazingly, the moment I boarded the bus I met someone – some crazy guy from New York who told me his life story; he had been a drug addict, had been in jail for violating his ex-girlfriend, but was now on his way of bettering himself.

More specifically, he was on his way of visiting his shaman in the jungle, and invited me to come along. I debated with myself; I was intrigued by the opportunity and felt that this was the real reason why I was on my way to this place, but had just met this guy and knew nothing about him or the shaman. My intuition won out… and these are the events that led me to this journey.

I have since also embraced all kinds of different practices that bring me into altered states – whether that's breath work or meditation. I also think nature is a major component – as is play, celebrating that inner child.

FINAL ADVICE: Wait for the medicine to find you. It'll find you when the time is right. And also, know that not everyone needs to take the medicine. There's no need to experience the medicine for the sake of experiencing it; but if you feel called to the medicine for healing, then yes. The bottom-line is that the medicine will find you when the timing is right and when you are ready

EDITOR'S NOTES:

KEY TAKEAWAYS FROM KATJA'S STORY

- These psychedelic medic
- ines are amazing tools for helping people heal old wounds and trauma, but many people also have truly transformational and spiritual journeys without experiencing any challenging moments (or exposure to old trauma) during their journeys.

- Many people experience spiritual awakenings and spiritual renewals when on a psychedelic journey – whether it's simply a deepening of spiritual values or experiencing a chat with God, the Creator, the Divine… or even alien beings.

- For many people, a psychedelic experience is truly life-transforming – and people often change/end relationships, switch careers/jobs, deepen their faith/spirituality, and broaden their worldview.

- In all sacred ceremonies – but especially those with mushrooms and Ayahuasca – guides and healers often use a ceremonial tobacco, which can be overwhelming to some people when taken in small spaces. Interestingly, tobacco is the most sacred of the Indigenous sacred medicines – used in virtually every ceremony as a means of connecting directly to the Creator; tobacco is most frequently used as an offering, either in order to give thanks, to make a request for wisdom or protection, or as a means of cleansing. (In the Indigenous culture, there are four sacred medicines: tobacco, cedar, sage, and sweetgrass.)

OTHER DETAILS

Katja Wallisch is a certified coach with a diploma in transformational coaching accredited by the leading global coaching organizations: the International Coach Federation (ICF) and the Association for Coaching (AC). She works with all types of people who want to transform their lives… through coaching, workshops, and retreats (with or without plant medicines). Learn more here: https://katjawallisch.com

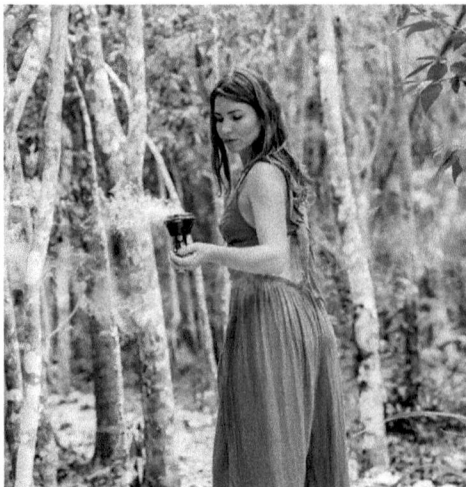

Katja during her Ayahuasca retreat.

CHAPTER TWENTY-ONE

Healing Story #18
Healing the Mother Wound with Mushrooms

STORYTELLER: Jessika, Female, BIPOC/Brazilian, Millennial

MEDICINE CONSUMED: Dried mazatapec mushrooms (most popular species of Magic Mushrooms)

DOSAGE: 5 grams

FOCUS/GOAL/INTENTION: Start to heal my relationship with my family - mother

BEST PART OF THIS JOURNEY: A deeper understanding of self-image/ how I viewed myself as a woman

BIGGEST CHALLENGE OF JOURNEY: Facing the pain of the abandonment wound related to my mother

....

PROFOUND HEALING JOURNEY STORY DETAILS

I've worked with mushrooms for many years now and they are by far the psychedelic that has changed my life the most on a personal and professional level. Mushrooms/truffles are very gentle in the way they show us our pain and always reconnect us with our own inner healing capacities.

I decided to go on a hero's journey after going through a very anxious week. During 3 days I did a preparation that included journaling and meditation. An argument with a close friend at the beginning of my week (as a result of thoughts and actions coming from a place of fear) was a determinant for me to decide to take a step further on my healing and go in silence and isolation for a few days.

After the journal exercise, I realized that the issues and troubling behavior patterns I've been facing today were not only a result of an abandonment wound or a mental health issue. My wounds go much deeper than that and by sketching a cloud of words on paper, I quickly concluded that I am in great need of healing my relationship with my family as a whole.

A big deal of pain was passed from generation to generation and I believe if I can manage to heal myself, I can break this chain so my future children won't carry the weight of their ancestors' unresolved emotions. This is work that I am willing to do for myself and them. And I am very conscious that this is not easy work. It's uncomfortable and unpleasant, but I no longer run away from sitting with all this discomfort because I know that's the only way, I can change this and live in a place of love.

The day of the journey came and so I prepared everything. In terms of music, I've used a curated playlist for this journey that I have worked with before (one set is called Heal, Play, Love by ACID FLORA, on SoundCloud). The mushrooms were home-grown, dried, and mixed into a tea with lemon using the Lemon Tek technique.

For set and setting, I had done a 3-day preparation with journaling and meditation and for the day of the experience. I chose comfortable clothing and created a cozy space in the living room with pillows, blankets, and candles.

I drank my mushroom tea.

As I closed my eyes to start my inner journey, my mind took me back again to Koh Phangan, Thailand, and other recent events of my life. I wandered through those for a few minutes but it was fast enough for me to notice that they were not where I was supposed to be going. I could then control my mind and bring me to the place where I didn't want to go: The place that I have been running away from for the past 10 years of my life.

I found myself in the house where I grew up, in Saquarema, Brazil. It was not like I was traveling through an old memory, but more like I was visiting the empty house. Very fast, then I felt why I didn't want to go there. Everything reminded me of the excess of control my grandma put into me and my sister during all the years we lived there.

I noticed how this control was present in every single detail of the house. I couldn't move the furniture without asking her, I couldn't even choose the blanket for my own bed. I couldn't spend too much time in my room or even lock the door. There was a way everything should be done, on her time and terms.

This lack of freedom was extremely repressive. I felt trapped in this memory of my house and a lot of pain took control of my body. I felt like a bird in a small cage, who never had the chance to use its wings to fly.

At the same time during this journey, I could understand why my grandma had such behavior, even though I don't know much about her history. She projected this control not only on us but probably did the same with my father when he was young. My mind went to my grandfather, Papi, the closest person I had as a father figure in my life.

My memories of him were carried off with a lot of guilt and sadness. I remembered how poorly I would treat him sometimes… a result of an anger that was not even directed toward him. I remember how he had his room separated from my grandma's. And of course, she chose where it would be and how it would be. Even him she would control.

I saw him sitting in his room, alone, and that made me sad. I remembered our last hug before he entered the ambulance when he knew we were never going to meet again. I apologized to him in these memories, for all the love I could not express back then. I understood his pain and hoped that he could understand mine.

My mind then took me to my father. I remembered his jacket that I kept for years in my closet because it had his smell. And then I remembered how with the years this smell slowly faded away. I couldn't go through many memories of my father, I guess because there was no pain or bad emotions I could relate to him. But he pointed me out to face my mother.

For most of my life, I blamed my mother for leaving us. I blamed her for not being there, I blamed her for who she was or who I thought she was. Having to face her on this journey was not something I wanted to do, but I knew I needed to do it.

But this took a different turn than I expected. I saw my mother but not as my mother. I saw her just like me, as someone who could be my best friend now, of the same age. I was shocked by how much she looked and acted like me.

I saw her as the 28-year-old woman that I am now and remembered she was almost 10 years younger than that when she had me. Suddenly I could understand how difficult it must have been to have kids when you don't know who you are or what you want in life. I saw her traveling around, always looking for fun and new experiences. Experimenting with drugs and sex with different guys, looking for something she probably didn't even know what it was.

I saw she was also on this ongoing journey of self-discovery and self-love. And she knew she wasn't capable of taking care of us because she didn't even know how to take care of herself. She was such a young woman then and she knew my grandparents would give us all that we needed, all the love. I think she felt a lot of pain once my father passed away and that might have been one of the reasons she couldn't face us anymore.

I saw so many similarities in her life, behavior, personality, and even looks. It was like a mirror. She was me and I was her. This inner work I am doing now. I believe she was trying to do it as well but somehow, she got lost in the process on the way – with the drugs and probably because of men. When I saw myself and her as one, I finally could understand and *forgive her*.

I could see her qualities rather than her flaws. I could even admire her for the beautiful woman that she was. And I could see why she was so well-liked by everyone and how much of her still lives in me. By seeing the beauty in her, I saw beauty in myself. By accepting her, I accepted myself.

And by forgiving her, I felt love for myself. When I was younger, my grandma used to say that I was just like my mother, but she would always use that with a negative connotation or when she wanted to make me feel bad about something. I didn't know how much that had influenced the ways I view my mother and even myself.

PROFOUND REALIZATION: Finally, I see, being just like my mother is something to be proud of. I love how I look, I love my personality, my social skills, the way I think, and my creative side. Finally, I realized that what was blocking me from embracing the woman I am and giving myself more love was the fact that I couldn't accept her and express love for her.

More than 2 years later, integration is still ongoing. I've had more journeys where the mother wound and my abandonment issues came up and a big part of my integration process has been to work in women-only spaces, journaling, inner child meditations, self-soothing, and grounding exercises.

This experience kickstarted my psychedelic path of working professionally with mushrooms and with women in women-only sacred ceremonies. I believe psychedelics can be extremely helpful tools to assist us in gaining a deeper understanding of our core wounds and having more compassion for ourselves and our parents.

KEY ADVICE: Don't journey alone (like I did), but request the assistance of a guide or tripsitter to hold space for you.

In terms of integrating, I regularly have had sessions of talk therapy for the past 2 years of my life, which also guides the integration of my psychedelic journeys.

PERSONAL BACKGROUND

I'm a BIPOC Brazilian woman who was raised by her grandparents and who faced a range of different traumas throughout my childhood and teenage years.

My quest for healing started with wanting to break myself from the limiting beliefs and negative thought patterns/ behavioral patterns I've had throughout my early 20s. I also wanted to improve my relationship with myself and my family, with whom it was always difficult.

Nowadays I work as an educator in the psychedelics space where I also do direct work with and for women. Besides that, I work in the Netherlands as a facilitator in group ceremonies and 2:1 psychedelic experiences with clients. Another part of my work is to also give extra support in preparation and integration as a coach.

I have a lot of experience with extraordinary states, ranging from breathwork to psilocybin, LSD, LSA, DMT, 2C-B (2C-B is a psychedelic drug of the 2C family, first synthesized by Alexander Shulgin in 1974), MDMA, ketamine, meditation, and trance states. Experiences in a healing/therapeutical context but also psychonautical and recreational ones.

Psychedelics have provided me ways to access subconscious material and also more of a somatic and holistic approach to healing. Talk therapy is limited, we go as far as we are ready to share. But psychedelics can go a few layers deeper, into the feelings and emotions, *breaking down some walls* we cannot easily reach through traditional therapeutic modalities

FINAL THOUGHTS: If the dose, set, and setting are well-thought-out and prepared, there is no such thing as a bad trip. Challenging experiences can arise but with the right support of a guide, people can navigate those and have deep insights into their psyche, giving them an amazing set of material to be worked with during integration. Most of the time challenges are actually related to our shadows, fears, or trauma.

EDITOR'S NOTES:

KEY TAKEAWAYS FROM JESSIKA'S STORY

- While set and setting are extremely important, taking time before a journey to detox, meditate, and find peace are important aspects of preparation for a psychedelic journey.

- A helpful technique for reducing stomach issues with consuming psilocybin involves mixing the mushroom with lemon... the Lemon Tek technique. This technique can shorten the journey's duration while also decreasing nausea, but it can also make the experience a bit more intense.

- Whenever possible, creating a private, safe, cozy, and comfortable "nest" for your journey is ideal. Hint: keep extra blankets around.

- Psychedelic medicines allow us to forgive the people who have hurt us (accidentally or with intent) and through that forgiveness, we can forgive ourselves – and enhance/expand our self-love.

CHAPTER TWENTY-TWO

Healing Story #19
I Encountered Jesus: My Burning Bush Experience

STORYTELLER: Charles, Male, White/Caucasian, Millennial

MEDICINE CONSUMED: MDMA with ketamine booster

DOSAGE: Heroic 500 mg MDMA; approximately 90 mg (exact dose unknown) ketamine

FOCUS/GOAL/INTENTION: Open to new experiences

BEST PART OF THIS JOURNEY: Feeling the infinite love of Jesus Christ

BIGGEST CHALLENGE OF JOURNEY: Coming back to the reality I faced, with people who did not understand

....

PROFOUND HEALING JOURNEY STORY DETAILS

My story begins about a decade ago.

I was living the life of an addict – and I thought it might last that way for however longer I might live. It's not the life I wanted to live, but I was deeply self-medicating with alcohol, cocaine, heroin, and benzos. I didn't understand it at the time, but I had serious issues with depression and anxiety, and I suffered with PTSD.

To be honest, this truly profound and life-altering experience was not something I planned… it just synchronistically happened the way it was supposed to for me. I took these heavy doses (as I typically did) to simply have a fun "trip." I started with the very high dose of MDMA (about 4-5 times higher than a typical dose) and just as it was beginning to hit me, I ingested the ketamine… then the journey roared into action.

The medicines hit me at once and I stood up and I looked at the people in my apartment and stated: "If I didn't know what the universe was about before, I know what it's about now. Wow."

I was just standing there in amazement. I realized that everything's made of energy; you've got positive energy and negative energy... I discovered that I'm so full of positive energy.

That's when I sat down in the chair and I looked around the room and everything just broke down to a quantum state. I could literally see all of the energy vibrating in everything in the room. That was when I realized that nothing is solid. Everything is made of energy. It's just at different frequencies and densities.

Then I looked up and there was this geometric portal-like opening above me; I felt like I was in a spaceship that all of a sudden skyrocketed into deep space. I was looking around and I could see all the stars and galaxies. Then, that's when I started thinking, "I'm dead. Did I die?"

I then looked down and noticed that I'm a being made of light, almost like in the movie *Cocoon*. Then, all of the sudden, there were some higher dimensional angelic beings – but they weren't angelic; they were more like amphibious beings. I began freaking out and again questioned whether I was dead or not. There was male and a female being, and the female came over to me and telepathically spoke to me, saying, "Charles calm down. Everything's gonna be okay." Then she gave me a hug and it was this beautiful hug; it was so comforting... It was kind of like she was my space mother or something. Regardless, I felt like I had known her for a long time.

Then this telepathic communication started where we discussed how we're all connected. *We're all one. The answer is love. Everything's going to be okay.*

All of a sudden, there was Jesus, and I went over and I put my hand on Jesus's arm – and it was an explosion of the most euphoric loving feeling that I had ever felt in my entire life. It was a feeling of ecstasy times a million – plus, there was Jesus and those extraterrestrial beings.

That was my **Burning Bush** moment; I had been agnostic up to that point. I lived my life on the things I experienced, not on faith. After this experience with Jesus, I can say I am much more spiritual.

I'll never forget that night. It was the most profound thing that's ever happened to me.

I had lived in fear my entire life, but because of this Divine experience, I knew from that moment on everything was going to be okay. The depression and anxiety were gone. I felt different than I had in a very long time. I was like a kid again. The release was so profound, like nothing I had ever experienced in my life… and yet I had no community to share the experience with.

The problems arose when I returned from my journey and the people around me looked at me like I was crazy. In fact, I had no one to integrate and share my experience; I actually began to feel more isolated from the experience because there was no one I could speak with about what I saw, what I experienced, and how I changed.

The sad thing is that I got the message telepathically that night that I was supposed to stop taking drugs. I was supposed to stop using alcohol – and I was supposed to heal myself. The reason given to me is that I was supposed to do all of this work because my mission in life is about helping other people.

I think if I would've had somebody to integrate this journey with properly that night, I might have gone in that direction. But the truth is that anytime I tried to speak about my experience with people, they acted like I was crazy. I decided my experience was way too "out there" to talk about with people who didn't understand it – and who couldn't help me integrate it.

The lack of community and the inability to integrate sent me to a place where I isolated even more. I almost became a recluse at that point, where I spent all my time online researching ketamine and experiences with DMT, watching *The Spirit Molecule* by Rick Strassman over and over and over again – because that movie was the only thing that gave me a sense that what I had experienced was normal.

EDITOR'S NOTE: *The Spirit Module* is based on the book by the same name. It's an investigation into DMT, a molecule found in nearly every living organism and considered to be the most potent psychedelic on Earth. DMT consistently produces near-death and mystical experiences, with many participants reporting encounters with intelligent nonhuman presences, aliens, angels, and spirits. Nearly all the participants felt that the sessions were among the most profound experiences of their lives.

I had to keep trying to convince myself that I didn't have to be freaked out by my experience. I might've lost my mind if it wasn't for his film, which is why he is one of my heroes. It was so comforting to know that I was not alone in my experiences.

After this experience, I also smoked DMT a number of times, with very similar experiences – except that I had a lot of oneness experiences – where I would go down to oneness with everyone and everything in the universe; in fact, the entire universe folded down on itself until I was in an entire place of oneness where I was alone – and I was everything.

On this one DMT journey, I was in the abyss of nothingness – and that was the night that I realized why we do this... because I basically was one with God, and I was God, and I was in the abyss of nothing all alone. It was lonely and it was scary because I was all alone – and I realized why we do what we do... because it's no fun being alone. Thus, we break ourselves down into the waters – or the droplets of water in the ocean of consciousness – and we put ourselves into one consciousness... and that's when I realized that I needed to take things a little bit lighter.

Still, I was alone in my journeys and alone in my integration. I had no community, and I relapsed into drugs and alcohol. I ended up getting completely strung out on heroin for a number of years, along with other drugs, such as cocaine and benzodiazepines.

It got to the point where my marriage had ended and I wanted to get sober and I wanted to get clean; that was actually one of the reasons why the marriage ended – because was I was so adamant about wanting to change my life and she wasn't ready to take that leap yet.

I remembered what had happened with my psychedelic deep dive experiences – and I knew I needed to get ahold of some DMT... so I could use it to get off heroin.

So I put the intention out there and the Universe delivered. I ended up getting my hands on some DMT – and that night I went into the journey with the intention of quitting heroin. During this journey, I ended up going to an alternate universe where there were all of these beings; all of them were gray... thousands of them. But then I noticed one different being; he was green and he was basically the one in charge of all of these other beings. He had a red ruby where his third eye would be – on his forehead. All of them were chanting and cheering for me and saying: "It's not too late! You can do it! It's not too late."

I knew they were speaking to me and I came out of the experience and I was crying and it really assured me that it was my time to stop the heroin. So I went over to my mother's house with some suboxone and locked myself in the bedroom. And I detoxed myself for about a week – and I ended up quitting the heroin.

I was still using alcohol, which of course always led me to using cocaine. So now, a few years later, I decided that I needed to quit the alcohol and I needed to quit the cocaine... So I did a deep journey with psilocybin mushrooms – about 6 grams. I locked myself in my bedroom in the pitch black, with a comforter over my head... and all of a sudden, I was being raised out of my body out into space – out in deep space – into the middle of the universe where not only was I out there but I became one with it.

I became one with everything in the Universe. I became one with God – and I was God. I realized that every time that I was taking cocaine or alcohol or any of these other bad substances – these low vibrational substances that were toxic for me – that I was basically poisoning God by my actions.

And it was a shell-shocking experience to where I came back to my body and I dropped to my knees and I was crying and I was looking up and I was apologizing to the Universe, to God, for everything I was sorry for doing – and what I had done. I knew at that point that I wasn't supposed to do those drugs and alcohol anymore.

My whole evolution with psychedelic medicines was a process. I had used them recreationally for a time – before using them for the therapeutic value – and every time I did use the medicines intentionally, I learned something new.

The truth is that the psychedelic medicines will show you what the answer is, but then you have to apply what you've learned to your life. All of my psychedelic experiences had led me up to this point – and the medicine showed me what I needed to do, but I was still self-medicating with these other compounds.

Interestingly, it was not until I actually used the ketamine protocol we use at our facility, where I went into my journey with the intention of taking myself to that next level of life, and to help me get through the depression and the anxiety – to the healing my neuropathways. The ketamine treatments we use are the inter-muscular shots, and the second time I did the treatment, I received a message that I no longer needed to do the medicine.

I was told I now was supposed to stop doing any psychedelic treatments – that I was supposed to be the walking embodiment of what the medicine can do for all the people who are still sick and suffering. I actually died – twice – during my ketamine treatments; not physically, of course, but I felt like I had just achieved this beautiful life... a fiancé, a young child, a new business. The message when I finally came back from the journey was that I wasn't dead and, wow, it made me appreciate everything in my life... that I had so much in my life I had been taking for granted.

During these experiences, I discovered my own divinity. I understood. Now it was my purpose to keep on manifesting my own reality and manifesting this healing organism that we have here today. The truth is that once you wake up to your own divinity, you realize that the only limitations we have are the ones we place upon ourselves.

I am now living out my purpose in life – or helping people live their best lives. I am divine, you are divine; everything is divine.

PERSONAL BACKGROUND

I was the sensitive kid growing up, never really felt like I fit in. I was fairly popular and had a lot of acquaintances; but still, I never really fit in to particular group. I was a good guy, but always making bad decisions.

I got into alcohol at a very young age. That led to cocaine and Xanax – and really anything I could get my hands on… eventually including heroin.

I do feel badly for getting in trouble with the law. I know it was embarrassing for my family and friends. Every arrest (possession, DUI) and almost every overdose or when I was sick from not using heroin… I had to go through these things. I had to go through the dark times so that I could become the person I am today.

I had crippling depression, anxiety, fear of death, and PTSD… but all these experiences help me relate to almost anyone who is hurting and seeking healing through psychedelic medicines.

Psychedelic medicines changed my life, along with integration, meditation, and a healthier lifestyle. Psychedelics totally reprogrammed my life.

Everyone matters. There is not one soul on this planet who is less worthy or deserving to receive these healing modalities. It is my mission to bring these healing modalities to the collective on a global level. I believe monetary status should not be what stands in the way of anyone's healing journey. We rise and heal together.

FINAL THOUGHTS: Psychedelics can be useful tools when done in a safe set and setting and incorporating integrative practices to assist you in the long term. The journey is not in the medicine, but when you take what you have witnessed and bring it back into a daily practice.

EDITOR'S NOTES:

KEY TAKEAWAYS FROM CHARLES'S STORY

- One of the most common tendencies of people suffering with depression and anxiety is to turn to either prescription medications or self-medicating with various drugs. Psychedelic medicines can rewire the brain in such a way as to help reduce these mental afflictions.
- While setting intentions is very important (as is having a safe environment), if the psychedelic medicine dose is high enough, a truly healing journey can still occur without set intentions, as this story demonstrates.

- Many people have truly profound spiritual experiences during higher-dosage psychedelic journeys; they often encounter God, Jesus Christ, angels, and other spiritual beings.

- Integration of these psychedelic journeys is absolutely essential – as is the community with which you share your experiences. Without integration and community, we can easily fall back into old and familiar patterns of self-destruction and addiction.

OTHER DETAILS

Charles is the Chief Education Officer and Brand Ambassador of My Self Wellness, a ketamine clinic located in Bonita Springs, FL. He and his partner, Christina Thomas, the president and founder of the center, invite anyone who is lost and suffering to their clinic for treatment. URL: https://myselfwellness.center/

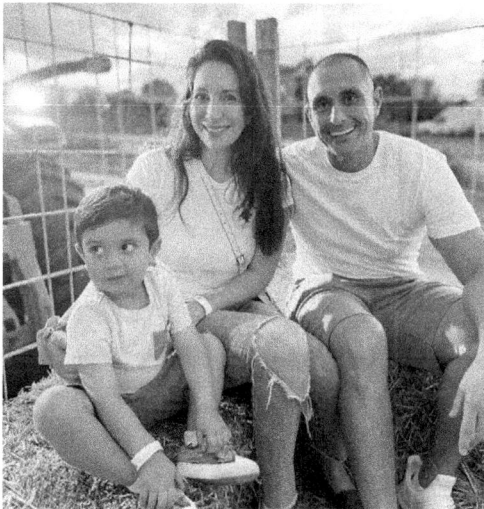

Charles and family

CHAPTER TWENTY-THREE

Healing Story #20
I Was Blind... But Now I See

STORYTELLER: Nirel, Female, BIPOC/Multiethnic, Millennial

MEDICINE CONSUMED: Ayahuasca

DOSAGE: 2 cups

FOCUS/GOAL/INTENTION: Love, trust, and surrender

BEST PART OF THIS JOURNEY: The clarity and grounded sober feeling the morning after, and integrating my journey with embodied mindfulness, feeling free in my authentic self-expression and creativity.

BIGGEST CHALLENGE OF JOURNEY: The subsequent months, a long-term relationship ending, more feelings of depression on the path of integration.

....

PROFOUND HEALING JOURNEY STORY DETAILS

I will share here about my first Ayahuasca journey, one of the most life-changing experiences of my life, and one of my many transformational psychedelic experiences.

A little over a year ago, I was with my partner at the time, who invited me to an Ayahuasca ceremony. I was in a dark place, mentally and emotionally, had been diagnosed with bipolar II (never on meds), general anxiety, OCD, and ADHD. I especially identified with the manic/depressive swings and chronic anxiety, and I felt open to sitting with the medicine.

When I said yes to Ayahuasca, I had no idea what I was getting myself into. I had never researched the medicine, I didn't know anything about it or what to expect, but that is how I like to approach life: without expectations, and without too much time before the experience to develop expectations or change my mind. So I agreed to sit with the medicine only about a week before the ceremony.

My diet was already mostly vegetarian, and I was not consuming alcohol (aside from an occasional glass of wine), so there was not much I did to prepare for ceremony other than what I had learned from a previous psychedelic experience, which is "love, trust, and surrender." So that's what I did, I practiced love, trust and surrender.

To this day, this is one of my life mottos, which feels so powerful with psychedelics and in life: *Love. Trust. Surrender.*

The ceremony was on Friday, July 16th. The address also had a 16 in it – my birthday number is 16, so it all felt like a sign.

The ceremony took place at a house in an urban area, in a medium-sized living room with about 25 people. The space was a bit uncomfortably crowded for me. But one of the walls was an enormous window looking out onto the garden. At night there would be a fire pit in the garden, so this window felt like a portal – to the sun in the daytime and the fire at night.

When my partner and I arrived, we settled in. We sat in our respective seats on the floor amongst the other participants, received instructions, and the ceremony began.

I drank my first cup of the medicine and waited. I don't remember each part of the experience in order, but will recount what stood out to me (not necessarily in chronological order)

I remember that as the medicine took effect, my body moved A LOT. In particular, I lay down and my hips swayed back and forth in rhythmic movements. This was meaningful to me, as I was bullied as a child and called "Big Hips." It took me years to have a positive relationship with my body and my sensuality, and this experience played a big role in the process.

I was shown a spiritual realm in which everything was perfect and nothing hurt; I didn't need to breathe, and I felt totally at peace. There was this profound sense of knowing that this realm I was seeing is the spiritual eternity – a timeless, formless present dimension, and then a realization that my physical body is just a host for the eternal soul.

In that space, I was reminded of the oneness, of connectedness with all beings. This concept has been a motif across my psychedelic experiences, and has informed how I view life: as one source of energy that inhabits individual beings.

GREAT INSIGHT: Life forms are all inhabited by this one eternal energy and so we are all one.

This timeless, formless present was visually dark. There was an alien quality to it: I remember neon green outlined visions of snakes and alien figures, moving very slowly all around. Like 2D sacred geometric and animal imagery, in 3D.

At some points I felt afraid – it was so comfortable for me to feel alive as this timeless, formless presence and feel that I was there, without breathing – that I feared I might actually die from not breathing. Of course this was irrational. I was breathing in those moments.. and would continue breathing. But it was interesting. I have had similar experiences during other psychedelic journeys, which feels related to the theme of resistance vs. surrender that has been such an integral part of my psychedelic journeys and life.

Some of the visions and insights I experienced involved sex, as a theme. I saw the concept of sex and the masculine/feminine dynamic as playful, with the masculine clearly desiring the feminine and the feminine enjoying being desired. I saw masculine and feminine characters dance, tease, and chase each other playfully. They made nonsense sounds – giggles and sighs from the feminine forms and groans and belches from the masculine. I saw the masculine as disgusting, which feels like it says something about my relationship with men at the time.

I received a download about feminine divinity – a message that we, as women, are powerful manifestors of our desires. As a woman who had repressed her desires for her entire adulthood (maybe life?), I felt shy during this Aya journey to accept the divine feminine power within myself. Women are socialized to be disconnected from our power. This conditioning, perpetuated by my relationship history with men, made it really hard for me to accept. The powerful, playful feminine creatures reassured me that I am one of them. They invited me to accept this reality. This Ayahuasca experience was a significant turning point in my journey, a call to embody my empowered divine feminine essence.

Throughout the trip, I came in and out. The medicine worked in waves, as psychedelics often do (at least in my experience), and I felt grounded every once in a while as I checked back into "reality." My partner was unaffected by the medicine, and I would check in with him once or twice, sneaking a brief hello or making eye contact. Once, when we did connect, I felt the weight of the traumas we had suffered together. The relationship involved so much turmoil, and I felt so, so sorry for my part in it. I had been so dissociated, and one of the greatest takeaways from this first Aya journey was, ironically, the sobriety it brought me – even if only temporary. The whole trip was like a wake-up call, coaxing me out of my dissociated, in-denial slumber.

One of the major themes of my experience was a call to accept reality, even if it's painful, and embody my authentic self. I saw a vision of my partner's mother, calling me to step into my authentic self. She asked, without words but rather telepathically understood, "When are you just going to be yourself?" Others appeared, in his family and in mine, as giant floating heads in the sky (not a gory image but a celestial one), encouraging me to just be myself.

At some point during the journey, I felt called to take a second cup. I didn't want to, but I felt called by the medicine, so I did. I thought I had already experienced a lot and didn't need more, but the medicine showed me I had more to see and to release.

I purged mostly halfway through and toward the end of the trip, from what I can remember. We each had buckets, but I did not use mine. Instead, I (get ready for the graphics) puked all over myself. I also went to the bathroom a few times throughout the night, twice accompanied by one of the women volunteers who was so sweet and stayed with me in the bathroom. In the morning, I puked again (this time into a bucket) and used the bathroom. I felt relieved.

I had the option to try Rapé (in ceremony) and Kambo (the morning after), but declined both. I felt it was enough with just Aya for my first time.

After this Aya journey, and also during another psychedelic trip on a previous occasion, the following phrase came to me: "I was lost, but now I am found. I was blind but now I see."

The morning after Ayahuasca, I felt a veil of fog had been lifted, clearing my mind. I now feel that my energy had been cleared. I felt so sober, so grounded in reality and in the present moment. I felt that my ego had been let go or set aside. I was covered in vomit, all over my clothes and hair. I was carrying around my teddy bear, which I had brought to accompany me during the ceremony. That morning, I felt the way I had imagined adults would feel – or maybe I felt the memory of what it felt like to be a child.

I felt so FREE. And light, like a weight had been lifted off me.

This free, light feeling lasted throughout the morning, as I exchanged life stories with people I'd met in ceremony. We had an integration circle that morning, in which we each shared about our experiences and ate a nourishing breakfast. Afterward, I went with my partner to his friend's house. When we arrived to his friend's house, I felt pretty good but tired.

Later, I felt sad and grumpy. I was triggered by something to do with my partner, and felt emotionally down. For the rest of the day I felt so-so. From what I remember, there was no significant short-term change. I went right back to the context in which I had been living: At my partner's parents' home with him and his parents, in a relationship that wasn't aligned, repeating destructive patterns, overworking, over- or under-eating, people-pleasing, generally unhappy and unfulfilled – yet in denial.

In the weeks after the ceremony, I felt more or less the same... until a couple of family trips. I visited my family twice in the months following, and the physical space, reflections, and conversations helped me see that I was unhappy in my romantic relationship and living situation.

IN TERMS OF MY INTEGRATION, IT HAS CONSISTED OF AN ORGANIC FLOW THROUGH:

- group mindfulness training (present-moment awareness without judgment)
- 3 months working with a spiritual coach 1:1 (childhood trauma, people-pleasing, resistance/surrender, procrastination, relationships, sex, my relationship with work, patterns)
- 2 months in one group coaching program (people pleasing/shadow work); 2 months in another (conscious communication)
- embodiment practices
- weights-based exercise routine
- healthy eating practices
- contact-beyond-contact dance facilitator training
- connecting with local and global community
- warm, supportive, accepting/celebrating and loving friends and family
- transformational festivals
- music (listening, creating & curating)
- voice activation
- meditation
- intentional time in nature
- loving my inner child, reparenting her, letting her run free
- self-care
- shadow work and shame/vulnerability work
- authentic creative expression through music creation and curation, visual art, dance and other performance and poems
- sharing healing practices that have helped me, with the intention of inspiring others
- relationships (more emotionally mature communication and dynamics in current and new relationships) and sex (conserving my sexual energy)
- dreams

- slowing down and relaxing more
- recognizing my mental conditions/diagnoses as symptoms, and working to uncover and heal underlying root traumas and other factors
- reading and re-reading transformational books (including, *The Power of Now*, *A New Earth*, *The Body Keeps the Score*, *How to Do the Work*)
- additional psychedelic experiences with various medicines, and subsequent integration
- volunteering for MAPS
- volunteering at a plant medicine retreat center with Ayahuasca and Huachuma (San Pedro)

In the time since my first Ayahuasca experience, I have undergone a massive transformation.

It has been one of the most change-oriented years of my life. My Saturn return is also coming up, which is all about major life change and embodying one's authentic or mature self, which also feels totally appropriate. Astrology is new to me but has resonated more than ever this past year.

Thanks to psychedelics and integration, this year has been a blessing: a year's worth of consistent practice to integrate several wake-up calls. I still feel hazy sometimes, but feel better equipped to come back to clarity time and time again.

In the past year, I moved across the country, ended my relationship of 2.5 years, ended my job of 1.5 years (and possibly my career of 5+ years), made countless new friends, reconnected with my family, discovered my passion for music, traveled, volunteered, facilitated healing and connection through content creation and event production, spent more time in nature and examined, considered and experimented with life from countless perspectives and styles.

PERSONAL BACKGROUND

I grew up religious until age 7 or 8, after which my family parted ways with the community and became gradually less connected to any concept of Source, God, or the Divine. I considered myself atheist, or agnostic.

Now, after my psychedelic experiences, I feel more connected to the Divine than in childhood. To me, it's all about a creative universal life force/Source energy, which is embodied in form, as humans and other life forces. We are all connected, we are all one, with all life and the Universe, with God. At least that is my perspective after these experiences, reaffirmed with each powerful trip.

Prior to my Aya experience, I had done consistent work to heal over the previous decade, practicing yoga, mindfulness, meditation and, in the 6 months preceding the Aya ceremony, talk therapy. I'd also had several other psychedelic experiences.

I felt so "lost" for the near-decade preceding my first Ayahuasca journey. Disconnected from my body, desires and needs, not knowing who I was, how I felt, what I wanted or even liked.

I oscillated between periods of depression and mania, felt empty, tried and tried to understand and treat my mental conditions, becoming more aware of my patterns but not knowing what I could do, blamed myself and internalized heavy shame for years, experienced chronic anxiety and generally checked out, not remembering conversations or events, not present.

Personal reflection: I now feel more aligned with my authentic self, and more honest with myself and others. I care less what others think about me or about what I do, am more compassionate with myself and others, and don't take things personally as much. I recognize my "mental disorders" as symptoms of underlying trauma and other factors, and practice self-care every day.

I am more discerning in my relationships, tuning into my intuition in my body in each present moment to decide how much energy to share with people or spend on a certain task or project. I am more aware of unhealthy patterns, feel better able to hold space for myself and others to heal, and know more wisdom and practices to facilitate healing. And I feel that I am a clearer channel for Divine creative energy to flow through, creating music, writing poems, and singing and dancing.

I am absolutely still learning and growing, and feel called to more healing experiences with psychedelics and integration. It is my intention to facilitate integration in community, as part of my offerings back to the community. I have also created and shared hundreds of video and photo posts, poems, songs, and podcast episodes inspired by my healing and spiritual journey.

FINAL THOUGHTS: I love to heal, grow, and connect – and love empowering and supporting others to heal, grow, and connect, too. And I am so, so grateful to these medicines, to healers, to the Divine. I am grateful for the traditional practices which integrate these medicines for healing and Divine connection, which have survived generations. I am truly so, so grateful. And it is my mission to share my experiences with others so that they may heal and connect and love and embody their authentic selves, aligned with the Divine, too.

Nirel is an embodied mindfulness coach, a music and event producer and DJ, and the founder/creative director at Get Grounded: https://getgrounded.life/. You can find her latest content and connect on Instagram @nirel_love , and listen to her podcast, Get Grounded, on Spotify, Apple Music and elsewhere.

EDITOR'S NOTES:

KEY TAKEAWAYS FROM NIREL'S STORY

- Integration is essential and encompasses many opportunities; yes to journaling and creative expressions; yes to community. But integration takes many forms – including taking better care of yourself by exercising, eating healthier, meditating, living stronger.

- The fear of not breathing – and thus the fear of dying from not breathing – is a fairly common psychedelic experience. Part of it is the ego's attempt to keep control of the journey. When you surrender to it, you can then move on to other issues in your journey.

- Negative narratives from our childhood often arise during a psychedelic journey, and are dealt with as the medicine tries to show you the truth… your truth.

- Psychedelics have the power to strip away the masks we often wear to hide our trauma, fear, and anxieties – as well as the masks we use to try and "fit in" – and show us our authentic selves.

- Integration can be accomplished in so many ways, as this story documents. The key to integrating is to just do it… and keep doing it. Integration of your psychedelic experiences is essential.

INSPIRING QUOTE "Psychedelics are not a substitute for faith. They are a door to authentic faith, born of encountering directly the sacred dimension of everyday experience. This is not the only gate to that discovery, but it is the most ancient and universal, and potentially the most accessible to the majority of the human race." – RICK DOBLIN, PH.D.

PART THREE: MICRODOSING

WHY MICRODOSING?

The goal with this book was to be concise, yet comprehensive... thus, a section on microdosing has to be included.

This section of the book is designed to provide you with an overview of one of the trendy areas of psychedelic medicine – using quite small (non-hallucinating) doses of the medicines to provide the many benefits of psychedelics.

Supposedly, entrepreneurs and tech giants in Silicon Valley have been microdosing for decades – to get clarity, direction, focus, and more.

You'll find one chapter that provides an overview of microdosing and then several stories illustrating the many benefits of microdosing.

CHAPTER TWENTY-FOUR

One Other Alternative: Microdosing

An emerging area within the psychedelic medicine field is the concept of microdosing – using very low dosages of a psychedelic compound to foster healing and transformation without having to experience a full-blown psychedelic experience one experiences with macrodosing the medicines.

More specifically, microdosing is the consumption of sub-perceptual amounts of a psychedelic medicine. With microdosing, you can get many of the benefits of the medicine without getting the "psychedelic" experience.

When microdosing– mostly with psilocybin or LSD – people report high levels of creativity, more energy, increased focus, enhanced relational skills, heightened spiritual awareness – all while reducing anxiety, stress, and depression. Most of the success stories with microdosing are self-reported and anecdotal, but more quantitative research is being conducted.

The idea behind microdosing is to encourage an increased state of perception and calm, rather than going into a hallucinating state. Thus, microdosing is taking a minuscule dose of the medicine… so small that you will not have any hallucinations or feel high.

Do you take daily vitamins or supplements for your health? Think of microdosing as a daily supplement for your spiritual and mental health.

As always, before attempting anything new, such as microdosing, do your due diligence and research and consult with trusted professionals before diving into the experience. Do NOT microdose if you are in crisis or if you are pregnant or breastfeeding.

" INSPIRING QUOTE "Microdosing involves consuming sub-perceptual doses of psychedelics – most commonly LSD and psilocybin – in a fixed protocol, like two times per week. Unlike "macro-dosing," microdosing is intended to integrate your psychedelic consumption into your daily routine to boost creativity, improve energy, increase mental focus, and enjoy better interpersonal relations." – PAUL AUSTIN **"**

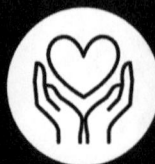

RESEARCH ON MICRODOSING

Interestingly, there was quite a bit of research conducted on microdosing LSD back during the first wave of psychedelic research in the 1950s and 1960s, but all that research was lost with the ban on psychedelics when they were moved to a Schedule I substance in the 1970s.

Happily, Dr. James Fadiman restarted the research and investigations into microdosing. He was convinced that microdosing with psychedelic medicines can have enormous psychological and health benefits with few risks.

Fadiman and his research team have collected thousands of stories about microdosing and found that people reported that they overcame their insecurities, anxiety, depression, and stress, as well as migraines, cluster headaches, and menstrual complaints.

Fadiman is known as the "Father of Microdosing;" beside his research of collecting stories, he also developed the most widely used protocol for microdosing, which is named for him: the Fadiman Protocol (consisting of one day on, two days off – for at least one month).

Fadiman also believes it's extremely beneficial to keep a daily journal to track observed effects and monitor well-being… thus, integrating the outcomes daily.

One of the most recently published studies on microdosing – and there have been few (and all with flaws) – found in the June 30, 2022, issue of *Nature: Scientific Reports*, states: "our findings of improved mood and reduced symptoms of depression, anxiety and stress are nonetheless generally similar in direction and size to the unadjusted small to medium positive effects reported [in previous research]."

Conversely, another of the current batch of research raises doubts about the impact of microdosing – beyond a positivity effect because participants were so excited about their microdosing. Published in the August 2, 2022 *Translational Psychiatry* journal, the authors conclude: "Clearly, more research is needed to decide whether microdosing with psychedelics can deliver at least some of its promised positive effects. This future research should also explore the potential impact of microdosing on aspects of human physiology that could compromise its long-term safety."

ADVANTAGES OF MICRODOSING VERSUS MACRODOSING

If you have ever taken a macrodose of a psychedelic medicine, you know much goes into the experience. First, there is the preparation – including diet, intention, and setting. Then there is the time commitment to the experience (including the recovery). Finally, there is the need to surrender to the medicine – to totally let the mind go where the medicine takes it. (For those who have not done psychedelics, surrendering is probably the hardest part for most people.

With microdosing, you:

- *Remain in complete control*
- *Have no hallucinations or visual effects*
- *Control the schedule – taking the microdose in the morning, afternoon, or even before bed*
- *Have low risks of having any mental or physiological reactions*
- *Can carry on with your normal daily routine*
- *Get to try psychedelics gently before deciding on a macrodose journey*
- *Have minimal commitment/changes required to diet, routine*
- *Can experiment with days on/off and dosage*
- *Do not have to spend as much time integrating, as with a macrodose*
- *Typically much lower costs than macrodosing*

FACILITATOR TIP When microdosing, experts suggest starting at the lowest dosage, gradually adding to it if needed to reach the desired outcome. Remember, though, that with microdosing, the effects will be subtle; do not push the dosage too quickly or too much.

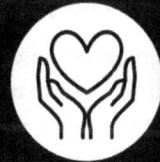

EFFECTS OF MICRODOSING

People report all sorts of positive effects from microdosing. From my personal experience, microdosing psilocybin left me in a more relaxed state, but never anything more than that. Microdosing LSD has been a totally different and much more positive experience. Again, find the medicine that works for you.

Anecdotal reports say some of the benefits people receive include:

- *Increased optimism, positivity, joy*
- *Sharpened focus*
- *Enhanced empathy and access to the heart*

- *Greater sense of openness, lightness*
- *Increased emotional and mental maturity*
- *Better levels of energy and productivity*
- *Augmented problem-solving*
- *Reduced anxiety, stress, depression*
- *Decreased negative self-talk*
- *Heightened sensory perception*
- *Deeper connection to authentic self*
- *Amplified creativity, mental alertness/clarity*
- *Decreased destructive tendencies*
- *Improved memory*
- *Lessened focus on pain*
- *Increased sense of spiritual connectedness/awakening*

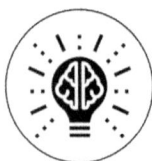

FUN FACT Microdosing has been a thing – a trade secret to innovation and creativity – in Silicon Valley for decades... with people stating that microdosing psilocybin and LSD help them think "outside of the box," as well as increase productivity.

HOW TO MICRODOSE

The key to microdosing is using the medicine in flights – though experts disagree about the exact timing. The reason for microdosing in this manner is to avoid building up a tolerance to the medicine.

The most common method is 1 day on and two days off (the *Fadiman Protocol*), with the idea that the first day you are at the full dose, the second at half (as the dose wears off), and the third is a break – before you start the regimen again. You could also try 4-5 days on, then 2-4 days off.

Another option recommended is one week on, then the next week off. Or the *Work Week Method* of five days on, two days off.

Whichever method you choose, most experts suggest sticking with it for about a month before making any changes to the dose or scheduling.

It also makes sense to start keeping a journal when you start microdosing, making note of feelings, concentration, creativity, etc.

Refer back to your journal and your experiences and in future months consider changing your dosage and/or timing.

As you move forward with your microdosing journey, you may eventually taper off completely, take a prolonged break, or simply microdose during specific times, as needed.

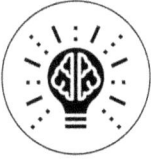

FUN FACT People microdose for all sorts of reasons – from healing trauma to easing anxiety to pain relief to increased focus and clarity to playing better at sports to learning new skills and languages.

MICRODOSING 101

Similar to taking a macrodose of a psychedelic medicine, it is important to follow a few guidelines so you get the most out of your microdosing.

1. DECIDE ON THE MEDICINE. While LSD and psilocybin are the two most commonly used psychedelics for microdosing, there's no reason you could not microdose with ketamine, mescaline, or MDMA. The key factor here is knowing the potential benefits of microdosing each medicine and then choosing the medicine that will hopefully give you the results you are seeking through microdosing.

2. BE CLEAR ON DOSAGE. Without question, you have to get the dosage right. Again, with LSD and psilocybin, the recommended dosages have been clearly identified through the research; with other psychedelics, you may have to rely on the community of users or a trial-and-error method of determining the best dosage. See the next section for full dosage recommendations.

3. DETERMINE DOSING SCHEDULE. The dosing schedule is probably the most discussed element of microdosing, but whichever method you choose, it needs to include days on and days off (to avoid building a tolerance for the medicine). The Fadiman Protocol is the most common method, but in reality, the best schedule for you can only be determined by experimenting and seeing what works best for you. In terms of time of day, most suggest taking the microdose in the morning so that you can feel the effects all day and not impact your sleep).

4. SET INTENTIONS. You must have a reason for microdosing – healing, clarity, energy, stress relief – so it's important to put that reason into a purposeful intention. Setting an intention of your goals with microdosing helps you be more goal-oriented and will be a key tool in determining if the microdosing is having an effect.

Some examples of goals/intentions for microdosing:

- *Enhancing relationships*
- *Finding clarity on purpose*
- *Solution(s) to challenging problem(s)*
- *Increasing self-worth*
- *Establishing a new habit*
- *Becoming proficient in a new skill*
- *Solving a complex problem*
- *Finishing building that app or website*
- *Healing old wounds, traumas*
- *Reducing anxiety*

5. JOURNAL/INTEGRATE DAILY. The cool part of microdosing is that you can incorporate the experience into a daily integration, monitoring any changes in feelings, thinking, moods, behavior, etc. Integrating and journaling can be done in numerous ways – with the key being using a technique that resonates with you.

6. REVIEW RESULTS AND ADJUST. Because so little research has been done with microdosing, it's essential for you to be your own test participant. Don't rush to judgment, but start reviewing the process after a month, reviewing your journal accounts and then make adjustments to schedule or dose accordingly.

DOSAGES FOR MICRODOSING

By definition, a microdose is a small dosage – designed to have an impact on well-being, but not enough so to have any obvious effects of "tripping."

Common dosages for microdosing:

- Psilocybin: 200 mg (.2-.4 grams)
- LSD: 8-24 micrograms (mcg)
- MDMA: 5-10 mg
- Mescaline: 10-40 mg
- Ayahuasca: 6 mg
- Ibogaine: 10% of full dosage

" INSPIRING QUOTE "I have felt different and I have been different. Whether it's the microdose, or the placebo effect, over the past month I have had many days at the end of which I looked back and thought... That was a really good day."
- AYELET WALDMAN, author of *A Really Good Day* **"**

MICRODOSING TIPS FOR BEGINNERS

Follow these suggestions for best results.

- *Follow a protocol and set a timetable for dosing*
- *Have a clear intention – and think on it daily*
- *Integrate daily by reflecting on the day and results*
- *Seek support if/when challenging aspects arise*
- *Include meditation, exercise into daily routine*
- *If possible, eat healthily – especially eliminating sugar, fried and processed foods*
- *Try to follow good, consistent, and healthy sleep patterns*
- *At completion, reflect on results and take a break before another round of microdosing*

EXPERT GUEST FINAL WORDS ON MICRODOSING

A MEDICAL PROFESSIONAL'S INTRODUCTION TO MICRODOSING PSYCHEDELICS

By C.J. Spotswood (aka "The EntheoNurse)

I am an advanced practice registered nurse (APRN) and board certified Psychiatric Mental Health Nurse Practitioner (PMHNP) with more than 20 years of psychiatric nursing experience. A large part of my nursing background and a significant influence on my practice was attending one of the 15 accredited holistic schools of nursing in the nation.

I have been writing and educating about the use of psychedelic medicines both nationally and internationally since 2018. Most recently, I became a student at the California Institute of Integral Sciences (CIIS) for the certificate program in psychedelic therapies and research.

When I was initially approached by entrepreneur and life coach Taraleigh Weathers (author of *How to Rock Your Life*) to partner with her for a microdosing program, I was hesitant and skeptical about microdosing, as all the research surmised that it was nothing more than merely a placebo response.

Intrigued, I dug into the research further… and became skeptical of the research. Realizing that people are going to microdose with or without my participation in this program, I thought I should do it if nothing else than approaching it from a harm reduction perspective. I dug deeper into the research on the classic psychedelics, chiefly psilocybin and lysergic acid (LSD), reading and reviewing as much research as I could – dating back to the 1950s.

It was interesting reading about microdosing before it was even known by this term; it was originally known as low-dose or threshold-dose in early publications.

I studied potential applications of these medicines, their pharmacology, and potential interactions, all the while compiling everything I learned into a handbook for the program I was conducting. This handbook eventually became what is known as *The Microdosing Guidebook: A Step-by-Step Manual to Improve Your Physical and Mental Health Through Psychedelic Medicine,* which was later published and released by Ulysses Press and distributed by Simon & Schuster in April, 2022 (on Bicycle Day nonetheless).

Since the time of publishing *The Microdosing Guidebook,* I have been privileged to have spoken with hundreds of individuals – sharing their personal stories and experiences of microdosing psychedelic medicines.

The most remarkable story was one that I learned about during my first public appearance after the release of my book. That day I met an older woman who told me about her husband's microdosing journey and recovery. Her husband had a history of vascular dementia and had experienced a stroke about 2 years prior, resulting in compromised use on the right side of his body. She explained to my wife and me how they were told that any hopes of improvement needed to happen within a year of the event and after that, the research has shown that further improvements are unlikely to occur.

After a year of working hard with his health care team, using conventional treatments that included various Western medications and physical therapy, he was fortunate to regain partial use, but not the recovery that they had hoped for. Shortly after, his mood and cognitive abilities deteriorated; he became more irritable and his wife was often the target of his frustrations, which was entirely out of character. Desperate and having heard about microdosing's purported effects, she spoke to his neurologist to answer the question, "May he benefit from a microdosing regimen?"

Deciding they had nothing to lose, she obtained a few chocolate bars online that contained 3.5 grams of psilocybin. She proceeded to break the chocolate bars into the precut 12 squares, then split them again. Each half square contained approximately 150 mg of psilocybin, the medicine he took every 4th day.

Weeks later, his mood improved, the irritability subsided, and she felt her husband had returned to her. She described, with tears in her eyes, how almost miraculously he regained near full use of his right arm once again. I, along with my wife, stood there with goosebumps on my arms and a tear forming in the corners of our eyes.

Now, I'm not saying his improvements are normal nor should they be expected, but this woman believed that microdosing brought improvements that she did not expect nor that were afforded by conventional medicines. This is just one story of hundreds that I have been told. Others described improvements in mood that have never been seen through standard treatments such as antidepressants and therapy. Improvements for what would otherwise be described as treatment-resistant depression, a term that I rather don't care for since most standard treatments are similar approaches, often antidepressants, working in similar manners, by increasing serotonin. Microdosing is different, acting on different serotonin receptors in the brain, which may account for improvements that conventional methods don't afford.

Microdosing still has some major hurdles ahead and one of the largest is the need to change the language of the laws across the globe. As it stands, psychedelic medicines are largely illegal, even in places that have progressed to decriminalize these substances; they are still illegal federally in the United States. In my book, *The Microdosing Guidebook*, I describe that while psychedelics are generally safe, especially when taken in microdose amounts, the biggest side effect may be what may occur if found in possession of these remarkable substances.

Other questions that I hope to be answered one day are:

- Can the dramatic changes seen as a result of taking macrodoses of psychedelics last longer as a result of microdosing?
- Can the pathways and growth that macrodoses afford be continued longer if a microdosing regimen is followed?
- Can we see improvements in other conditions as a result of microdosing… such as improvements in chronic headaches and the management of physical pain? (The initial research shows that it can.)
- Can microdosing improve other neurological conditions such as Alzheimer's, head injuries and traumatic brain injuries (TBIs), or Autism? Time will tell.

While we wait for these answers, I still question if people are reporting such amazing healing effects and dramatic changes as a result of microdosing. Why is this happening? Can we really reduce it down to being nothing more than a result of the placebo effect? Should we even care?

I question what the researchers are missing and further, do they really know what they are looking for? To this day, the biological causes and effects of mental health and psychiatry are not completely known, so how can we be so quick to dismiss what is not understood?

CHAPTER TWENTY-FIVE

Microdosing Story #1
Researching the Power of Microdosing: Yes, It Works!

STORYTELLER: **Danielle, Female, White/Caucasian, Millennial**

MEDICINE CONSUMED: Psilocybin Mushrooms

DOSAGE: 130 mg (.13 gram)

PROTOCOL/SCHEDULE FOLLOWED: Stamets… 4 days on; 3 days off

FOCUS/GOAL/INTENTION: Prove to myself whether microdosing works or not

....

MICRODOSING STORY DETAILS

While I had done much healing through macrodosing (large doses of) psyche-delic medicines, I did not become interested in the concept of microdosing until working on my master's thesis. I knew of the power of macrodosing, because of my personal healing, but I was very skeptical about microdosing.

During the master's program, I decided to start experimenting with microdos-ing psilocybin mushrooms. My intention for experimenting was to prove that microdosing wasn't therapeutic, and in order to heal with psychedelic medi-cines, large doses are needed – that is where my head was at.

Going into my microdosing journey I did not yet know the tools to gain deeper healing with this medicine, and I was very busy, so I did not have much time for self-reflection. About a month into my microdosing journey, it was seemingly doing nothing, and I was starting to think I was right. I thought to myself "yep. It's bullshit; the microdosing did nothing."

I stopped microdosing, and then after about a week, I was walking with my dog and all of a sudden, I had this severe fear. I had suffered from anxiety pretty much my whole life and, interestingly, that's something the large doses of psychedelics never helped me with. One of my intentions for macrodosing, especially with Ayahuasca, was to overcome my fears and to live with courage, but it never lasted for me. Macrodosing helped me heal many traumas and significantly helped me make better life choices, but anxiety still lingered.

Sometimes the anxiety was so intense I wouldn't want to leave my house because I was certain something bad was going to happen. Not to me, but to my beloved dog, Anicca, who is my love. I've known him for 10 years and he has been such a blessing in my life. I felt a need to protect him. There were even some days I couldn't go outside, or if I was outside, I was in a fear state the whole time, filled with paranoia.

So... after a week of not microdosing, I was walking my dog and all of a sudden fear washed over me – with a sense that something bad was going to happen. In that moment, I realized – "whoa, I haven't had this feeling for a month. Wow. Okay."

After that experience, I started taking microdosing more seriously and I decided that I was going to investigate microdosing in greater depth, and more consciously. It was very humbling that week – and I apologized to the mushroom spirit: "oh my gosh, I'm so sorry mushrooms; you're small but powerful. Okay, okay... I'm going to start working with you with intention and with respect." When I first started microdosing, I didn't go into it with respect – I went into it with doubt and a lot of ego.

This is how I learned what tools can be used to gain deeper healing while microdosing, and I teach my clients these tools of how to microdosing with intention. It took me a year of experimenting on myself to really figure out what works and what doesn't work while microdosing.

This medicine brings to the surface what needs to be healed, and then it helps you gain more clarity and allows for different perspectives while navigating through the difficult emotions, or memories that may arise. There are tools to help with this navigation, such as journaling, meditating, and being in nature. The key is having that space for yourself, so that you can witness your past traumas with eyes of healing and love. It helps you see different perspectives and it gives you that space in order to make different choices.

Now I am able to share these tools with my clients. Also, I am a person who can hold space for my clients to encourage self-reflection and realizations during their microdosing journey. Having someone to talk to while microdosing, who can be that clear reflection for you, is important. Many folks don't know how to hold space, so when you're sharing your experiences they may judge them, or put their personal opinion on your experiences and realizations.

I love the mushrooms because they're gentle. Mushrooms say, "Hey let's look at this over here. And ooh this may be a little hard, but don't worry – we're gonna come over here and it's gonna be all blissful. Okay, this might be a little difficult, but it's all good. I've got you."

That's been my experience with mushrooms. And I feel like the microdosing has really enhanced and strengthened my relationship with mushrooms so much.

PERSONAL BACKGROUND

I had a pretty traumatic upbringing. Before getting into it, I want to make clear that it wasn't all bad. My family did love me and wanted the best for me, in the way they knew how. I love them all very much, and absolutely want no harm to be done by sharing my story.

I was disassociated (and didn't know it) up until I was in my early twenties. I realized that I didn't have any memories of my childhood, and I would be in a conversation and suddenly wake up in the middle of it – not even knowing what I was talking about. That's just how my brain was, and how I survived. I realized in my early twenties something was wrong. So, that's why I started exploring spirituality, and started a meditation practice. I wanted to be present, and to get my memories back.

When I was a teenager, I cut myself, and when I was a child, I had thoughts of wishing I didn't exist. I was raised with a lot of emotional abuse; I wasn't allowed to have a voice, and I felt like my existence was a nuisance, and that I was unwanted. I also had a lot of physical ailments; I couldn't digest food well, and I found out in my early twenties that I had Celiac disease. That added to the emotional pain of my childhood, because no one took my illness seriously, not even doctors – I was hurting so badly.

I used to think I was ugly and fat. I was never fat in my life, but when I was about age eight or nine, I would steal my mother's diet pills and would take them because I thought I needed to lose weight, which I think may have led to digestion problems. I was blessed to be raised around nature, and with animals. Being in the forest would bring a deep sense of peace, and I always connected to animals; sadly, my animal friends weren't protected – and they often got hurt or killed.

I started experimenting with psychedelics 21 years ago when I was 14. I started with mushrooms, but they were too strong, too powerful for me; I didn't have the tools to heal with them yet. Later on I preferred LSD because it was a more fun experience for me.

Besides psychedelics, I tried many harmful substances – I tried really hard to get addicted to them, but apparently my spirit was too strong.

I tried a lot of things to hurt myself, including recklessness, driving the car way too fast; it's amazing I'm not dead. I also liked going to rave parties in San Francisco. I would get into cars with strange people, when everyone was high on ecstasy. (I did ecstasy a lot when I was a teenager.) I did all these things to help me escape from my reality of pain and suffering.

Today, I feel so blessed to be alive and to be healthy. I feel blessed I didn't go down that path of self-destruction and addiction, and that I didn't end up on the streets, or doing things to permanently hurt my body. I recognize that I'm still not feeling completely comfortable in my body, because I still do things to change how my body is feeling, such as drinking coffee or eating unhealthy foods when I am feeling uncomfortable. That's still something I'm working on; we're all healing from our childhood trauma, right?

I was introduced to working with psychedelics with intention in my mid-twenties; primarily I was introduced to Ayahuasca in Brazil, which was life-changing. And from there, I worked with San Pedro (also known as Huachuma), and I shifted my relationship with LSD and with mushrooms to work with intention while macrodosing. Working with high doses of these psychedelic medicines, along with integrating the experiences, has provided profound healing for me.

This is why I previously thought that macrodosing was the way to attain deep healing, not microdosing.

When I was writing my thesis at Humboldt State University, I interviewed 18 people using in-depth interviews about their experiences and motivations with psilocybin mushrooms. Through those interviews, I heard a lot about microdosing. I'd never microdosed and I thought microdosing was bull-crap. I thought it was a placebo at best. I believed the big dose was where the healing happens – that's where my mind was. But like any good scientist, I decided to start experimenting on myself.

After that initial experience with microdosing mushrooms, I've also microdosed with LSD and with San Pedro – all separately of course. It is important to honor each medicine, to fully understand the teachings they provide. I haven't microdosed San Pedro in a while, but I am going to start microdosing with this medicine again. I have to be ready, because for me, the medicine is very intense. When microdosing San Pedro, I can't take a microdose and just go through my day, because it brings so much to the surface. I need to be in nature and just sit with it. For me, it was a lot of family stuff coming to the surface – seeing those family cycles and personal cycles so clearly.

Microdosing LSD, on the other hand, is a bit more superficial for me. I am not saying anything bad about LSD – it is a very deep, very spiritual medicine that should be treated as a medicine. LSD, of course, has been misused and I hope that in the future the fear will dissipate from this medicine, and it will be taken as medicine, and in ceremonies – just like San Pedro and mushrooms are used in ceremony.

In terms of microdosing protocols, it takes a little bit of experimentation to find what feels most supportive for people. I suggest when someone is trying to taper off of SSRIs, working through something big, or experiencing severe depression and anxiety, to microdose every other day. Every other day is more balancing, and the medicine is still doing healing work in your brain the day after. For others needing even more support, especially with tapering off of certain medications, I suggest two days in a row, with a one-day break. I found that to be quite helpful for my clients. Also, for some people getting off of prescription medications, it may be helpful to microdose every other day, but do so taking two doses in that same day; for example, one in the morning and one in the evening.

KEY ADVICE: Remember, microdosing is a personal journey, so take the time to experiment with what feels most supportive for you and your needs.

Normally, I tell people to start with the Stamets Protocol because I respect Paul Stamets. He has been doing this for a long time, and his protocol – four days on, three days off – has been showing great benefits, so that's what I generally recommend. I also tell people to pay attention to that third day off; if that third day off finds you extra irritable or you're feeling extra depressed, then it may be better to switch to every other day for a more balancing effect.

After you have been microdosing for a few months or longer, I recommend taking breaks from microdosing to see where you are at – even up to a month or a month and a half break. For me personally, I stop microdosing until I'm feeling anxious, and then I start microdosing again. It's been a very cool journey because in the very beginning, it took a week of me not microdosing, and I'd feel anxiety again. And now, I can go a month and a half until I start feeling that anxiety creeping back in. Eventually what's going to happen is there will be no more anxiety, because this medicine truly heals the brain. Healing takes time, and patience.

Psychedelics have been banned for 50+ years, which has been a great disservice to our mental health, but sometimes the greatest healing comes when we emerge from places of darkness. The last 50 years have been very dark. People have suffered – and continue to suffer – and many are taking pharmaceuticals that are just not working for them.

Many people are feeling overwhelmed and some are having suicidal ideation, feeling powerless to do anything. Now that psychedelic medicines are emerging, people are truly being able to heal, after years and years of living a life of misery. People are able to emerge from the darkness into a place of balance and light, and I love how much more powerful these medicines are for healing because of this.

Danielle is a microdosing coach, and is the founder of Microdosing Humboldt. For the last 10 years, she has studied psychedelic medicines, along with personally benefiting through intentional therapeutic exploration. Her website is Microdosing Humboldt (https://www.microdosinghumboldt.com/)

EDITOR'S NOTES:

KEY TAKEAWAYS FROM DANIELLE'S STORY

- Whether macrodosing or microdosing, it is extremely important to go into these experiences with full knowledge, proper planning, and true respect for these medicines.

- A key part of integrating your psychedelic experiences is finding/discovering the insights from the medicine – and then acting on those insights – that's a big part of integrating your experiences and manifesting them into your life.

- Besides its uses for healing, microdosing is also a great tool for helping people wean off poorly performing prescribed medications, such as benzos and antidepressants.

- Microdosing is also a great way to get introduced to a psychedelic medicine – allowing a gentle introduction (with no hallucinations) – before considering a full macrodose journey.

CHAPTER TWENTY-SIX

Microdosing Story #2
Microdosing for OCD and Anxious Attachment

STORYTELLER: Marina, Female, BIPOC (Mexican/Lebanese), Millennial

MEDICINE CONSUMED: Psilocybin (Golden Teacher)

DOSAGE: 100 mg (2x daily)

PROTOCOL/SCHEDULE FOLLOWED: 5 days on (weekdays), 2 days off (weekends)

FOCUS/GOAL/INTENTION: Distress Tolerance and Acceptance

....

MICRODOSING STORY DETAILS

I embarked on my healing journey in 2020 as someone living with Obsessive Compulsive Disorder (OCD), Anxious/Disorganized Attachment, and PTSD.

Psychedelics helped me lift a veil of hopelessness that gave me a chance to create new neuropathways and disrupt the catastrophizing looping that occurs with OCD.

My story of healing begins when I first started taking prescription Zoloft in conjunction with trying different modalities of therapy, including Cognitive Behavioral Therapy (CBT), Somatic Therapy, Hypnosis, Traditional Talk Therapy, and Group Distress Tolerance classes.

Zoloft assisted with reducing obsessive loop cycles, however I often felt numb, experienced digestive issues resulting in an ulcer, and it greatly impacted my sex drive. I was then prescribed Wellbutrin to offset the side effects.

Following a therapy session one day, I decided to partake in a psilocybin macrodose session by myself. I noticed that it allowed me to look at my situation from a wider perspective and not tainted by the trauma lens and nervous system response that often limits my ability to fully process the situation. The biggest thing for me during this experience was my ability to meet myself with compassion rather than judgment or shame.

This was HUGE for my personal healing. This single experience has had the largest impact on my healing to date. Following this experience I made the decision to slowly wean off my SSRIs and begin to practice transformational microdosing.

I began researching the clinical studies that had taken place surrounding psilocybin and OCD. I attended speaker events such as the Psilocybin Conference, read *How to Change Your Mind*, as well as the Netflix docuseries based on the book. I also viewed the documentaries *Dosed* and *Dosed 2*.

I joined forums such as the Sisters in Psychedelics (SIP) and the OCD & Psychedelic Support group hosted by the San Francisco Psychedelic Society to connect with others. It was during this time that I discovered both Mycology Psychology and Microdosify as suppliers – and had great experience with both.

Mycology Psychology is a woman-owned business that connects you directly to someone to conduct an evaluation of your needs and provide recommendations of which product is right for you and explains the protocol. They also promote transformational microdosing – and I felt very connected to their brand. They recommended 5 days on (weekdays) and 2 days off (weekends), which is the protocol I follow to this day.

In the beginning of microdosing, I had a lot of emotions arising – emotions that had been in a purgatory state on my SSRIs. However, the looping cycling lasted only 2-3 days – versus weeks (and in some cases months) in the past. After navigating that experience, I've since noticed I meet myself with a lot more compassion rather than the shame and judgment I typically experience that feeds the OCD looping cycle.

MY MICRODOSING BENEFITS: Besides helping with my OCD, I also noticed an increase in my mood with day-to-day activities, heightened sensory awareness, and a major increase in my productivity, both professionally and personally.

I also practice breathwork with some cold-water exposure (Wim Hof Method), in addition to specific guided breathwork meditations focused on inner child and trauma healing. I make sure to make time for play, hobbies, and passions.

In the past, I was so serious about how to heal "right." I was so highly focused on all the work to be done/problems at hand, that I neglected the simple joy of play and passion. Not only did it rob me of fully living my life, but it also exacerbated the issues as it was the OCD showing up in another form.

I practice radical self-love and distress tolerance when heavy feelings arise and meet myself with more gentleness when I digress, which in turn allows me to not stay in stuck cycles.

Part of my wellness routine includes regular physical activity and volunteer work within the community. Finding community, I feel, is a huge part of healing. It reinforces that we do belong, we are enough, and that nothing is inherently wrong with us. Meeting other neurodivergent mountaineers and rock climbers is incredibly inspiring to me.

My first year of healing pre-psychedelics was rooted in an obsession to cure my OCD and never get triggered again – another attachment to perfection.

My second year of healing has focused on radical self-love, acceptance, and embracing my shadow. The introduction of psychedelics, helped with rewiring my brain to make these shifts more possible… being able to view things through a wider lens and show up with more compassion in the process.

I believe my quality of life will continue to improve with transformational microdosing and embodiment practices.

My tips for anyone considering psychedelics is to do your research and have realistic expectations. If you're currently on medications, you need to be aware if they are compatible with psychedelics. Know your condition; not every mental health condition is created equal – and psychedelics may cause psychotic breaks for certain disorders.

Psychedelics are not a happy, cure-all substance that will change your life requiring no work on the user's end, but when you put in the work (including intentions and integration), psychedelics can make a major impact.

KEY ADVICE: While bringing things to the surface is beneficial to help process and move forward, it is important to mentally prepare yourself with realistic expectations of what the journey may entail.

PERSONAL BACKGROUND

Being a child of divorce as a Highly Sensitive Person (HSP), I developed anxious attachment. This resulted in my mother having to stay in classes with me in my early childhood.

I noticed violent and religious obtrusive thought cycles as young as six years old. I become obsessed with being "pure of thought," which fueled the obtrusive thought cycle and resulted in the debilitating feeling of guilt and shame. I became obsessed with reassurance-seeking from my mother. I felt the need to confess any potential bad thought, terrified that she'd no longer love me if she knew the "true" me.

In my early teens, I began searching for my symptoms, already having an idea that I must have *Pure O*, a specific obtrusive thought-based type of OCD. However, even though I thought I might, I still believed my thoughts defined who I was. It wasn't until researching that I learned more details on how looping occurs with OCD and passing thoughts do not indicate truth. In one support group a therapist said, "If you tell yourself over and over again not to think about white elephants, it will be the first thing that comes to mind." That simple statement was a huge part of my healing process.

Education on my neurodiversity has helped me eliminate almost all of my obtrusive thinking. The last ongoing part of my OCD I continue to navigate is Relationship OCD – related to my anxious attachment as well as guilt and distress tolerance during traumatic events like death or breakup.

I believe therapy, hypnotherapy, somatic therapy, and now psychedelic therapy has all had its place.

Traditional therapies helped me in times of major distress, such as loss from suicide (and murder) and heartbreak as well as help me understand tools to utilize during events of extreme distress.

Psychedelic therapy has allowed me to use those tools in times that it has felt debilitating, or my judgment has been clouded by my trauma. Psilocybin isn't a magic pill (just like conventional modalities aren't), but I noticed I'm able to strip away my limiting perspectives that go into fight or flight when facing triggering events.

Instead, I'm able to sit with the discomfort, which allows me to ultimately process it and move forward. Does it mean I will never get triggered again when I process the discomfort? No, but it helps rewire my brain – showing me that it is possible to sit with it and it will pass. This has been a huge breakthrough for well-being.

FINAL THOUGHTS: One of my biggest breakthroughs was with macrodosing – and being able to access my trauma with the tools provided in therapy – but tap into a wider spectrum that allowed me to feel deeper compassion and understanding for my own vulnerabilities. I think there are many benefits for macrodosing, but I believe transformational microdosing is more sustainable to create lifelong change, and can be complimented by a series of guided macrodosing journeys.

EDITOR'S NOTES:

KEY TAKEAWAYS FROM MARINA'S STORY

- Prescription drugs, especially those used for depression and anxiety, tend to numb or mask the underlying issues causing the disorder; they do not address the underlying issue.

- One of the hallmarks of psychedelic medicines is that they allow you to see that underlying trauma/hurt from a lens of safety and with compassion – not shame, fear, or guilt.

- Many people are now microdosing as a tool for weaning themselves from the pharmaceutical tools used for depression and anxiety, including SSRIs and benzodiazepines.

- Prescription medicines typically list many side effects, adding to the dangers of using them, including an increase in suicidal ideation. Psychedelics, on the other hand, have minimal (and only temporary) side effects.

CHAPTER TWENTY-SEVEN

Microdosing Story #3
Dipping My Toes Into Microdosing –
and Finding Healing

STORYTELLER: Kristin, Female, White/Caucasian, Gen X

MEDICINE CONSUMED: Psilocybin

DOSAGE: 100 mg – 200 mg

PROTOCOL/SCHEDULE FOLLOWED: Intuitively led with 5 days on;
2 days off for 3 months. Then, a 2-week break, followed by 150 mg 4 days
on 3 days off for 3 months – with deep journey work laced in between.

FOCUS/GOAL/INTENTION: Heart-centered healing from trauma and a gentle
introduction to the medicine

....

MICRODOSING STORY DETAILS

As we record this call, I noticed the date – and it is exactly the year anniversary
of my microdosing birth-day!

I started my journey with true psychedelic medicines by microdosing first, and
it was a gentle introduction to the beautiful medicine of psilocybin. Microdosing gave me the ability to create a relationship with the medicine in a way where
I gained trust.

That trust was beautiful because I was healing; I was able to be more in the
present; I was becoming a better mom, breaking old patterns. Through microdosing, I was able to connect not only to myself, but also to my children in such
a different way. I was able to push aside that default mode network (DMN) and
pause, check-in sometimes in situations that were difficult – and see things from
a different perspective.

With my trauma-filled background, trust is a huge thing – and one that I've been learning to rebuild. I've also been working on my root chakra for a long time. My heart center has a few blocks, but it's very open.

Before I tried microdosing, I did have one ketamine session, and I remember it popping me out of my depression for a little bit. I also tried equine training because I was still searching for what was home for me – my dharmic path—what am I meant to do.

My first microdosing was such a lovely experience. I come to tears thinking about the way my heart felt so open and connected. I took 100 milligrams first thing in the morning with no food.

Within about 40 minutes I felt a slight shift. I went outside and stood looking at the sunrise. I breathed in and felt more at home in my body than I had in a long time. Microdosing is amazing and also a bit difficult, because even with a microdose, things do come up. It's like you throw a big rock in a pond and all the muck that has settled down through the years and been forgotten is awakened to be seen and worked through – and then it settles back down and it's clear.

Each time a "rock" gets thrown in, through this healing process the settling time gets quicker and the pond continues to clear up. When I work with clients as a microdosing practitioner some don't like that feeling and they want to quit. So many of us are used to numbing out or disassociating. Microdosing psilocybin doesn't allow for that. The medicine wants you to be able to work through it and release so that you can be more clear and more connected to self, to nature, to others, and to source.

My intention at the time was an introduction to the medicine, but also healing. I actually was very depressed at the time and I was going through a really rough moment of my life; it was post-divorce. I was a single mom with three kids, and then there's this battle going on with the trauma that happened earlier. It was still so hard. And as far as my parenting goes, I was struggling so much with my kids; and they were also struggling because their dad wasn't around anymore – except every other weekend. Add that covid was still hanging around. A lot of stressors going on.

With all this stuff going on in my life, I decided to start microdosing while I was at equine training. I'm without the kids, and I remember the first time I took the medicine, I was also doing yoga (I had been doing yoga ever since I had received my yoga teacher training), and I remember breathing and I felt this connection to my heart that was different; I could feel it – and I knew it wasn't placebo; I felt it – even as I breathe right now – just a deeper connection to my heart. I will always remember it – and it was simply a microdose of the medicine.

I have also found that the experience varies, depending on the mushrooms used. For me, personally, the really sun-shiny mushrooms like the Gold Caps, or the Golden Halos and the Golden Teachers – those actually create something like that of an energetic antenna for me, and with kids around, it increases my input and I actually get increased anxiety… so those intensify whatever emotions I'm having at the time.

I have found I relate much better to other mushroom strains, such as Ghost or Penis Envy – at least when I have my kids around. They tend to be a little bit more dense and keeps me more grounded.

My experiences with microdosing – and all my training – then led me to offering these things to my clients.

My microdosing success and comfort and trust then allowed me to consider a macrodose.

FINAL REALIZATION: I have all the tools I need for healing.

In terms of integrating, I had been trained so thoroughly that integration is the number one thing that's important – so that even before I started microdosing, the idea of integration had already been implanted in my head. The medicine is great, but if you don't integrate, then you've done nothing pretty much.

I went into my microdosing practice knowing integration was going to be key and it became part of my mission from those initial moments, which led me to create a book I use in my practice (and available on Amazon and elsewhere): *Integrate: 3 Month Microdosing Guide.*

PERSONAL BACKGROUND

I grew up extremely orthodox – Mormon Orthodox; I mean people wouldn't call it that – they just say that you're really Mormon. I used to be really that; I was so religious. They have a term called *Molly Mormon* for women or *Peter Priesthood* for men, and I literally felt like I was Molly Mormon. I was so excited to be so good and keeping all the rules, living the commandments.

I felt really happy and good and safe doing that, but Mormons also have a health code – and part of that is about eating vegetables and fruits and eating foods during the seasons and not consuming drugs of any sort – so, for example, we didn't consume coffee or green tea or black tea. I grew up not even being allowed to drink Coke or Dr Pepper, and I remember in high school feeling guilty about drinking those sodas. So, for me, there was shame behind what I would consume and how I lived my life.

That Mormon upbringing kept me from exploring things until I was 44 years old. Suddenly, I decided I was done. I decided that I was thinking for myself from here forward. So the deconstruction of all those years indoctrinated with those rules had been quite intense. But I also retain some good memories and experiences, like a missionary trip to Paraguay.

Since 2016, I personally have been on this pathway of helping others be able to break through the trauma, to be able to get out of their heads; I called it "get out of your mind get into your life."

I went to Mount Shasta for Reiki attunement (the process by which a person receives the ability to give Reiki treatments). I was led to Mount Shasta due to my desire to connect to the root chakra of the Earth, which I know sounds kooky and a bit woo-woo, but I had been studying yoga and been shifting my religious perspectives and turning more to spirituality.

So I was led to Mount Shasta to get a Reiki attunement, and while I was at there, I heard (inside of my mind), "Welcome home Kristen I love you. This is for you."

This experience helped me release a lot of fears that had been built around thinking for myself and branching out from a religion that I had grown up in – and also being more open-minded to new ways of seeking out religious and spiritual experiences.

While I was at Mount Shasta, I discovered that the Reiki master was also a shaman – and he mentioned that they were going to be offering a ceremony in the near future, using either psilocybin or Ayahuasca. His partner mentioned that psilocybin was more gentle than Ayahuasca – and that was the catalyst for me to be more open to the medicine.

As I drove home from Mount Shasta – through California and Oregon and all those beautiful redwood trees – my dear friend and I discussed our plan to ultimately have a macrodose of psilocybin to help us heal from the deep trauma that had occurred to both of us in the same year.

Interestingly, even though I was able to get the magic mushroom in my possession fairly soon after our return, I never felt like it was the right time. And honestly, I had a little bit of fear of diving deeply into the medicine without somebody to be with me and to guide me through it.

I focused on practicing Reiki and having Reiki clients, but I soon started feeling I was meant to work within the medicine realm; that I was meant to be a guide – even though I hadn't even worked with the medicine yet.

So I sought out training and I was led to a group that's actually based in my state in Salt Lake City: Salt City Psychedelic Therapy Training Program (SCPTTP).

I decided that I would do the program – and this way I could learn and be able to use the principles to do my own work for my own healing while I'm going through the training. We were being trained by MAPS professionals, by James Fadiman, and other professionals. During the train, they kept mentioning microdosing and all of the benefits for neural plasticity.

I had personally been on a mission for myself to learn how to be more in the present moment – and while the instructors were talking about the benefits of microdosing, I just instantly knew this was my calling. And that's the path that led me to finding mycology psychology, and being called to become a practitioner with microdosing.

My background is in health education and then I did some postgraduate work in positive psychology. I'd already been speaking and working with mindset and practices – micro-practices I would call them – gathering tools together to be able to be in the present moment.

So all of my life had been preparing me to take the next step, which was adding to my tool belt the plant medicine and the microdosing. Once that was accomplished and I felt called, it was time for the macrodose.

It was in April. My brother convinced me that it made sense, if I was going to macrodose, to go for it in a big way so I could break through all my barriers… and so I did, with 8 grams. I did this heroic dosage on my own. I had the training – and – I also had established a relationship with the mushroom. I also felt very called to do this macrodose on my own so that I could go completely in without even being concerned about anyone else's well-being or what they might think of me during my journey.

I call my experience my *Jedi Mind Fuck*. The medicine was a teacher and it was deep – and at the very beginning I was told, "We've prepared you for this. Are you ready? You're going to learn things you haven't ever learned before. Here we go." And then I was just deep in the medicine.

But, interestingly, it'd also bring me out, saying "Okay, let's take care of you. Let's go get some water. Let's go to the bathroom." And so I got up and I took care of myself physically.

And as soon as I returned to the sofa, the medicine would take me right back on to the journey.

To be honest, I still have some challenging days – even with consuming the medicine. Parenting is always something challenging for me, along with dealing with my ex, who is a beautiful but very flawed man – hurting and making bad choices. That said, the medicine has helped me to be able to handle life – and my gifts have been more augmented my increased mental abilities. (I was getting so foggy from the medicine I take for epilepsy.)

I just had this interesting experience – and the medicine does send you messages. So just yesterday – with my daughter who is four years old – she was throwing this fit, this very primal experience where she is hitting and wanting to bite me and all these things. To avoid her antics, I went to a closet for a moment; I'm sitting in the closet and I look up and there's this box and it says "old patterns" on it. And I was like no way!! Oh my gosh. It was my mom's box of old sewing patterns, but I'm sitting there in the closet expressing my gratitude for the message. Then I exited the closet and approached the situation with my daughter with a new strategy. It was truly a breakthrough moment for me – and it's all because of the work I have been doing.

FINAL THOUGHTS: I think the most beautiful thing that the medicine has given me is the opportunity to see that there are so many paths and that every day I get to choose. Every day I get to decide, and every day I get to make the moment my moment – and in my moment, I choose love… and I choose my heart.

As I say in my microdosing practice, with microdosing, you have all the control. Unlike other uses of psychedelics, microdosing is a safe container for consciously working through inner blockages, past trauma – including PTSD and CPTSD – and other areas you need to create within yourself. Microdosing is also highly therapeutic for creative blocks, connecting with your body, and accessing higher states of consciousness.

EDITOR'S NOTES:

KEY TAKEAWAYS FROM KRISTIN'S STORY

- There are multiple natural healing modalities – meditation, yoga, Reiki, equine therapy, acupuncture, massage, sound therapy, hypnosis, breathwork, psychedelics – and your goal is to find the one(s) that work best for you.

- Microdosing a psychedelic medicine before undertaking a macrodose is a great way to learn about the medicine, develop a relationship with the medicine, AND receive healing and other benefits through intentionally microdosing.

- One of the major and unexpected benefits from ingesting psychedelic medicines that researchers are just now discovering is what seems to occur in the brain. For reasons to be determined by researchers, these medicines seem to help the brain reconnect lost pathways, as well as create new ones – something referred to as neuroplasticity. (Experts now believe that the negative thought patterns that occur with depression could be the result of interrupted or impaired neuroplasticity processes – and psychedelics seem to help "rewire" some of these patterns for improved mental health.)

- Ketamine, which is not a traditional psychedelic – it's classified as a dissociative medicine and is better known for its use as an anesthetic – is showing remarkable results for a number of conditions, including: pain, depression, PTSD, OCD, chronic migraines, fibromyalgia, and anxiety.

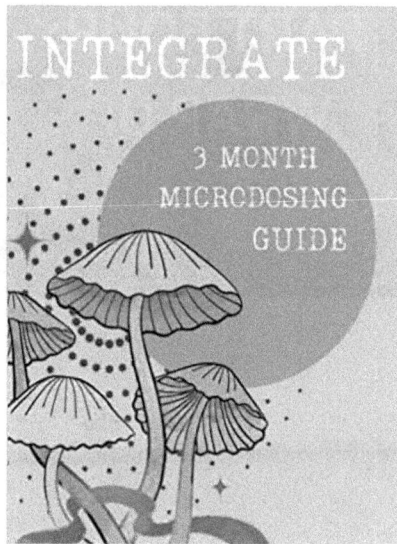

Kristin's workbook for
integrating microdosing.

PART FOUR:
WRAP UP

CHAPTER TWENTY-EIGHT

Key Takeaways for Your Psychedelic Journey –
Summary/Conclusion

Where does all this information, all these transformational stories, leave you? What have you witnessed with the accounts and details in this book? Do you feel a calling to psychedelics – to one of these psychedelic medicines? What medicine is calling you the most? And if you are feeling a calling, are you pondering a macrodose journey or microdosing? As you look ahead to joining this psychedelic revolution of healing, what method looks like the best fit for you?

While all the stories in this book are individual events, unique in every aspect, they are truly representative of the amazing discoveries and healing taking place right now! Yes, you need to be physically and mentally stable, and you really should prepare with a social media/news blackout, and you need to eat cleanly and exercise, but these are all important steps to your healing.

In order words, these psychedelic medicines should just be ONE part of a complete wellness makeover of your life. But before we go there, let's wrap up the learning we have gained from the previous chapters.

> ❝ **INSPIRING QUOTE** "I am convinced that psychedelics are not a panacea, but they can play a role in healing and connection, both for the people that choose to use them and for those that do not." - MATT ZEMON ❞

PSYCHEDELIC MEDICINE STUDY RESULTS

Research using psychedelics as a potential healing modality has exploded over the last five years, with studies and trials being conducted around the world at leading universities and cutting-edge psychedelic companies.

All medicines/drugs approved for use by the FDA must go through several phases of trials before making it through to approval. Phase 1 trials are all about safety of the potential medicine; Phase 2 trials, sometimes split into Phase 2a and 2B (relating to finding best dosage), focus on the efficacy of the medicine treating a specific condition. If the medicine satisfactorily passes the first two phases, the final stage, Phase 3, is a large trial, typically with 100+ participants; and the results must show conclusive evidence that the medicine being tested is more effective or safer than the current medicines being used for the condition.

Many psychedelic medicines are being tested in a variety of drug trials, with both MDMA and psilocybin the closest to moving to FDA approval.

In terms of the medical conditions being studied with psychedelic therapies, here's the list (from most studies to least):

- *Depression*
- *Treatment-resistant Depression*
- *Post-Traumatic Stress Disorder*
- *Suicidality*
- *Addiction*
- *Bipolar Disorder*
- *Anxiety*
- *Alcohol Use Disorder*
- *Pain*
- *Palliative Care/Cancer*
- *Headache Disorders*
- *Eating Disorders*
- *Obsessive-Compulsive Disorder*
- *Postpartum Depression*
- *Opioid Use Disorders*
- *Fibromyalgia*
- *Autism*
- *Smoking (Addiction)*
- *Traumatic Brain Injury*

Learn more in this article:
https://www.lucid.news/psychedelic-medicine-beyond-ptsd-depression/

In terms of some of the most exciting research – that is pushing everything, from excitement about the healing potential to potential changes in how some of these psychedelics are classified – here are some of the most promising that came out around the time of this book's publishing.

MAPS PHASE 3 TRIAL WITH MDMA FOR POST-TRAUMATIC STRESS (PTSD)

As discussed elsewhere in the book, MAPS has been leading the way with MDMA research.

In this most recent trial, two months after treatment ended, 88% of those who had received the MDMA therapy continued to see a reduction of their symptoms by at least 50%.

More astounding: 67% of those who received the MDMA treatment improved so much they "no longer met the diagnostic criteria for PTSD."

Rick Doblin, Founder and Executive Director of MAPS, believes this data to be so positive that MDMA therapy to treat PTSD will be legalized as soon as 2023.

PITFALLS TO HEALING The biggest challenge most people experience when taking one of these psychedelic medicines is surrendering to the experience. The mind wants to stay in control, but for true healing and transformation, you must truly and completely surrender... perhaps even using that phrase as a mantra while under the medicine: I surrender.

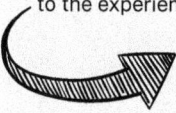

AWAKN LIFE SCIENCES PHASE 2 TRIAL WITH KETAMINE FOR ALCOHOL USE DISORDER

Awakn is a biotechnology company researching, developing, and commercializing therapeutics to treat addiction with a near-term focus on Alcohol Use Disorder. Earlier this year, it published the results of the Phase 2 trial attempting to treat Alcohol Use Disorder in 96 patients.

The company found that 6 months post-treatment, 86% of those treated with ketamine therapy remained abstinent from alcohol, compared to just 2% who were abstinent before the trial began.

Furthermore, the rate of relapse was 2.7 times lower than for those in the placebo group.

The company announced plans to move to a Phase 3 trial, though the start date is not yet known.

COMPASS PATHWAYS PHASE 2B TRIAL WITH PSILOCYBIN FOR TREATMENT-RESISTANT DEPRESSION

Compass Pathways, a mental health care company dedicated to accelerating patient access to evidence-based innovation in mental health, recently announced the start Phase 3 trials – following the success the company found in the Phase 2b study. The people being studied are those with a severe form of depression who have tried other standard treatments that have failed to help them.

The 2b study found that a single 25 mg dose of psilocybin, in combination with psychological support, was associated with a highly statistically significant reduction in depressive symptoms after three weeks, with a rapid and durable response for up to 12 weeks. More specifically, more than one-third (36.7%) saw a decrease in their symptoms by 50% or more – and 29.1% of these patients improved enough to enter remission.

JOHNS HOPKINS STUDY COMPARING PSILOCYBIN TO SSRIS FOR MAJOR DEPRESSIVE DISORDER (MDD)

This follow-up study follows several previous studies by Johns Hopkins Medicine researchers that demonstrated that psychedelic treatment with psilocybin relieved major depressive disorder symptoms in adults for up to a month.

In a follow-up study of those participants, the researchers report that the substantial antidepressant effects of psilocybin-assisted therapy, given with supportive psychotherapy, may last a year for some patients.

The Johns Hopkins Center for Psychedelic and Consciousness Research is an undeniable leader in psychedelic research, backed by $17 million of funding. Researchers are studying the potential of psychedelics for illness and wellness: to develop new treatments for a wider variety of psychiatric and behavioral disorders with the aspiration of treatments tailored to the specific needs of individual patients.

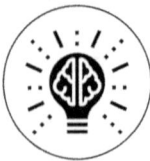

FUN FACT The word entheogen comes from Greek origins, with entheos for divine and genesthai for generate – and refers to a connection with the sacred, the inner divine; it's commonly used when the psychedelic medicines are taken with spiritual intent or when they have spiritual effects. They include LSD, Ayahuasca, psilocybin, mescaline, Ibogaine, DMT.

MIND MEDICINE'S PHASE 2B TRIAL WITH LSD FOR GENERALIZED ANXIETY DISORDER (GAD)

This second trial is just getting started. The Phase 1 clinical trial demonstrated the rapid, durable, and statistically significant effects of LSD to safely mitigate symptoms of anxiety and depression. The results of the Phase 2b trial will guide the dose selection and development strategy for the pivotal Phase 3 clinical trials.

GAD is a chronic, often debilitating mental health disorder that affects approximately 6% of U.S. adults in their lifetimes. Symptoms of GAD include excessive anxiety and worry that persists for more than six months.

The Phase 2b trial in patients diagnosed with GAD is a multi-center, parallel, randomized, double-blind, placebo-controlled, dose-optimization study. The trial plans to enroll 200 participants to determine the reduction in anxiety symptoms 4 weeks after a single administration of the LSD.

MindMed is a clinical stage biopharmaceutical company developing novel products to treat brain health disorders.

PSYCHEDELIC MEDICINE 101

The most important takeaway from the work in this book should be that while these psychedelic medicines show enormous potential for upending our knowledge of mental health therapies and transforming our (mis)use of antidepressants and anxiolytics, that we consumers must be proactive and diligent in conducting our own research before diving into the deep end of psychedelics.

These medicines are not a cure-all, nor are they suitable for everyone. The medicines do work independently in your brain, building new neural pathways and connections, but the emotional healing and transformation comes after the medicine – when people have to do the work of integrating the insights and healing into everyday life. And, for some people with mental and physical health conditions, these medicines – at least at the macrodosing levels – are not recommended.

So, the first step should be determining if one of these psychedelics is a good fit for you – for what you want to accomplish, given your mental and physical health conditions. This part of your preparation is critical. One great tip here is finding and building a community who will help guide and support your efforts, pre- and post-experience.

The second step should be deciding on the best protocol for taking one of these psychedelics. Microdosing is a growing field within psychedelics (with more research coming) that offers many of the benefits from psychedelic usage without having to deal with the hallucinating components of macrodosing. Macrodosing is the protocol that offers you the full psychedelic experience.

The third step is determining how you will partake in the medicine; you have several options. If you are interested in ketamine, you can likely find a clinic near you; these clinics are completely legal. You can attempt to find and join one of many clinical trials being conducted on psychedelics; this method is the safest and most legal. Or, you could attend a sacred ceremony at one of the legal psychedelic churches or travel to a retreat in a country where the medicine is legal.

Or, you could find one of many underground centers/ceremonies where a facilitator guides you on your journey; these centers are underground because of the illegal status of the medicines. Finally, you could undergo the whole experience on your own (or, ideally, with a tripsitter if ingesting a macrodose), sourcing the medicine from a reliable (but not legal) source – or by growing/harvesting your own.

The fourth step is preparing for an intentional psychedelic experience. This step should include a move to healthier living and eating, an avoidance of negative situations and people, a plan for reducing the use of any meds (under medical supervision) that may negatively affect the use of psychedelics, and determining the proper set and setting.

The fifth step is starting your protocol – either the full-on macro-journey or your microdosing journey.

The sixth step is documenting and integrating your experiences. As so many people state in their stories here, after consuming psychedelics you change – but, sadly, the world remains the same. You need to find a way to live your new and better life in a world that remains unchanged and indifferent. Additionally, you need community – people who will listen to your stories and who support your journey… people who get you now that you have transformed. Community can not be emphasized enough; you need supportive people to sustain the changes you will need to make in your life.

The seventh step is deciding next steps – but only after fully integrating your first experience. Options here include being done with psychedelics; attempting a different dose or protocol with the same psychedelic medicine; or trying a different psychedelic or psychedelic combination.

FINAL PSYCHEDELIC MEDICINE TAKEAWAYS

Each person's experience with psychedelic medicines is utterly unique – whether with macrodosing or microdosing. Our body chemistries, brain functioning, and overall health mix with a particular dosage of a certain medicine – leading

INSPIRING QUOTE "With psilocybin, we discover that we do not have to look outward toward the futile promise of life that circles distant stars in order to still our cosmic loneliness. We should look within; the paths of the heart lead to nearby universes full of life and affection for humanity." – MICHAEL POLLAN

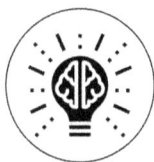

to unique experiences, some of which will be truly profound – while others may be more subtle, but no less transformative.

The key to remember is that these medicines are tools for your overall health and well-being. They can help you overcome stumbling blocks that you had no previous awareness existed – showing you what needs healing, what needs your attention, how to live a better and more spiritual life. But you need to find the medicine that works best for your condition – and for you – and then find the right protocol and dosage that works best for you. You need to be intentional in your work… you need to set clear intentions, surrender to the experience, and integrate any lessons learned.

Why should you consider finding healing through psychedelic medicines? As the stories in the book show – and which is backed up by numerous academic research studies broadcasting the breakthrough status of psychedelics – here are just a few of the highlights from intentionally consuming psychedelic medicine:

Psychedelics are poised to have a place in the future of how we treat many mental health and wellness issues. These medicines connect us with our truths, show us what needs to be seen, and help us feel and experience and react to past traumas and events buried deeply in our psyche. We come through these experiences dramatically changed – we're stronger, healthier, and more purposeful in all we do.

Set & Setting are vital components of the intentional use of psychedelic medicines. Your mindset – intentions and expectations and preparation – and a safe and comfortable setting for the journey.

Integration is essential. These medicines are powerful tools for healing, including emotional and spiritual growth. We have to be committed to integrating all the things we saw and learned in our psychedelic experiences – and putting them into action, truly incorporating all these lessons into our lives… moving forward in healing, personal growth, and spiritual connection. Integration needs to be done through self-reflection and deep thinking – as well as being part of a "psychedelic" community that understands and supports your psychedelic experiences.

Psychedelic medicines can aid healing with just one experience – as long as set, setting, and integration are properly and thoroughly done. These medicines are not addictive, but some people do experiment with the different medicines to discover the one that best works for them.

Microdosing, an effective tool on its own, is also a good way to gradually introduce yourself to a psychedelic medicine – to gain trust and comfort in the medicine, without the worry of having a full-blown psychedelic journey (until you want one).

THE PSYCHEDELIC EXPERIENCE

APPENDIX 1:

Psychedelic Organizations and Web Resources

Some great organizations here – with all sorts of resources, from the latest scientific breakthroughs to finding clinical trials to tips on all aspects of the psychedelic medicine experience. Listed alphabetically.

ATLAS OF PSYCHEDELIC RESEARCH: a great tool for discovering research on psychedelics happening around the world. Jointly developed by Blossom, the University of Lisbon, and Synthesis Institute. *URL: https://atlasofpsychedelicresearch.com/*

BECKLEY FOUNDATION: a nonprofit whose goal is to create a future in which the therapeutic potential of psychedelics is widely recognized, medically applied and harnessed as a tool to heal, increase well-being, and study consciousness. It has been at the forefront of global drug policy reform and scientific research into psychoactive substances, and actively collaborates with leading scientific and political institutions worldwide to design and develop ground-breaking research and global policy initiatives. *URL: https://www.beckleyfoundation.org/*

BLOSSOM: is focused on making information about the potential of psychedelics available to all stakeholders to help speed up the psychedelic transition from trials to practice. Users can search for information on psychedelic papers, companies, key people, news, events, and more databases. *URL: https://blossomanalysis.com/*

BONFIRE: Focused on integration and community, this group offers monthly online meetings to help guide and support people in the community. For people looking to do more serious work, it offers the "Campfire Crews," which are facilitated groups with a guide or therapist to help support each member's growth and healing. Meetings are a combination of structured discussions and activities. *URL: https://www.bonfire.earth/*

CENTER FOR PSYCHEDELIC & CONSCIOUSNESS RESEARCH: from researchers at Johns Hopkins University, one of the leading universities in the psychedelics space, where researchers focus on how psychedelics affect behavior, mood, cognition, brain function, and biological markers of health. *URL: https://hopkinspsychedelic.org/*

CHACRUNA INSTITUTE: a nonprofit that promotes reciprocity in the psychedelic community, and supports the protection of sacred plants and cultural traditions. "We advance psychedelic justice through curating critical conversations and uplifting the voices of women, queer people, Indigenous peoples, people of color, and the Global South in the field of psychedelic science." *URL: https://chacruna.net/*

COSMIC SISTER: "champions women's frontline voices, emphasizing our responsibility – as Earth's apex predator – to rapidly evolve from a cultural and behavioral perspective. We advocate for the right to journey with sacred psychedelic plants and fungi to jump-start rapid cultural evolution, starting with women's healing, empowerment and self-liberation." *URL: http://cosmicsister.com/*

DECRIMINALIZE NATURE: a nonprofit that believes plants should not be illegal. Its mission: "improve human health and well-being by decriminalizing and expanding access to entheogenic plants and fungi through political and community organizing, education and advocacy. Its vision: "We envision happier, healthier individuals and communities reconnected to nature and entheogenic plant and fungi traditions and practices." *URL: https://www.decriminalizenature.org/*

DOUBLEBLIND MAG: a biannual print magazine and media company covering timely, untold stories about the expansion of psychedelics around the globe, stating: "Our stories strive to reach everyone touched by psychedelics, not just the loudest or most influential voices." It also offers a variety of affordable online classes with some of the leading psychedelic experts. *URL: https://doubleblindmag.com/*

DRUG POLICY ALLIANCE: a nonprofit with a mission to end the war on drugs – and especially drug users: "We believe that every person should be able to work, parent, be housed, have a community, experience joy, and live freely regardless of drug use." It seeks to advance policies that "reduce the harms of both drug use and drug prohibition, and to promote the sovereignty of individuals over their minds and bodies." *URL: https://drugpolicy.org/*

EMPATHIC HEALTH: its mission is to craft the best healing community in the world for its members, and to have fun doing it. It is a peer-supported psychedelic integration community that connects like-minded people to learn, share, and help others. *URL: https://www.empathic.health/*

ENTHEOGENIC RESEARCH INTEGRATION AND EDUCATION (ERIE): a nonprofit organization dedicated to the sharing of entheogenic and transpersonal knowledge. It also hosts peer integration circles to facilitate meaning-making and community building, as well as monthly educational events – including symposiums, forums, and conferences on varied topics surrounding entheogenic research and activism. *URL: https://erievision.org/*

EROWID FOUNDATION: a nonprofit educational and harm-reduction resource with an amazing library of resources – 60,000 pages of online information about psychoactive drugs, plants, chemicals, and technologies – including entheogens, psychedelics, new psychoactive substances, research chemicals, stimulants, and more. Its mission is to provide access to reliable, non-judgmental information about psychoactive plants, chemicals, and related issues. *URL: https://www.erowid.org/*

ENTHEONATION: a web show featuring visionaries pioneering the cutting-edge of awakening through psychedelic science, modern shamanism, and new paradigm lifestyles. Its mission: "to provide informative content about the therapeutic benefits of psychedelics & visionary plant medicines in a way that integrates science, culture, & spirituality. We love exploring non-ordinary states of consciousness for personal, spiritual, and social transformation." *URL: https://entheonation.com/*

FIRESIDE PROJECT: a nonprofit that operates the Psychedelic Peer Support Line, providing free, confidential emotional support by phone, text message, and mobile app (firesideproject.org/app) to people who are having psychedelic experiences and people who are processing past psychedelic experiences. The support number is 62-FIRESIDE (623-743-7433), open every day from 11am to 11pm PT. *Everyone is welcome by the fireside. URL: https://firesideproject.org/*

FUNGI ACADEMY: a global community of mushroom cultivators, psychedelic explorers, permaculturists, and eco-changemakers – working together to empower individuals and cultivate deeper connections through revealing the magic of fungi. It works to make mushroom education accessible and easy by connecting a global community to empower the growing and sharing of fungal wisdom. *URL: https://fungiacademy.com/*

GRADUATE STUDENT ASSOCIATION FOR PSYCHEDELIC STUDIES: focuses on supporting collaboration among graduate students, recent graduate students, and post-doctoral residents who are engaged in psychedelic research and clinical practice. *URL: https://gsaps.org/*

HEFFTER RESEARCH INSTITUTE: a nonprofit organization that promotes research of the highest scientific quality with classic hallucinogens and psychedelics (predominantly psilocybin) to contribute to a greater understanding of the mind leading to the improvement of the human condition – and to alleviate suffering. *URL: https://www.heffter.org/*

HEROIC HEARTS PROJECT (HHP): a nonprofit organization with a mission to build a healing community that helps veterans suffering from military trauma recover and thrive by providing them with safe, supervised access to psychedelic treatments, professional coaching, and ongoing peer support. It connects military veterans struggling with mental trauma to psychedelic therapy options including Ayahuasca, psilocybin, and ketamine. *URL: https://www.heroicheartsproject.org/*

H.O.P.E. PROJECT: offers four-month programs that connect military spouses, female veterans, and Gold Star wives with counseling services, support and community – all around psychedelic healing journeys. *URL: https://the-hope-project.org/*

LIGARE: an open network of people who desire legal and safe access to psychedelics – who believe that Christianity and other existing religious traditions offer paths for preparing, experiencing, and integrating mystical experiences, including those served by sacred plants and compounds… to gain widespread acceptance of psychedelics as a tool for emotional, physical, and spiritual well-being. *URL: https://www.ligare.org/*

LUCID NEWS: with a mission to provide informed, honest, and transparent journalism that covers the growing integration of psychedelics into society and their broad implications for human wellness. – offering news and opinion from a wide range of perspectives to help readers navigate this pivotal moment of innovation and transformation. *URL: https://www.lucid.news/*

MELANATED CONSCIOUSNESS: a nonprofit organization that evolved from a passion to connect with like-minded Black and Brown people having psychedelic experiences. It was created to support women – who have made sacred medicines a part of their practice for healing and transformation. Also about connecting BIPOC individuals with BIPOC facilitators. *URL: https://www.melanatedconsciousness.org/*

MICRODOSING COLLECTIVE: a nonprofit dedicated to leading the conversation about the necessity of legal, regulated, and safe access to microdosing, while educating on the benefits of legalizing microdosing psychedelics for optimal human wellness… research-backed, community-driven, and rooted in evidence-based outcomes. *URL: https://www.microdosingcollective.org/*

MICRODOSING FOR HEALING: is a nationwide community of diverse individuals committed to the intentional practice of microdosing earth medicines. Ranging in age from 21 to 91, community members come to practice for physical healing, emotional balance, mental health, spiritual discovery and personal growth – learning cultivation skills, best practices, personal development and reverence for natural medicines within a warm, welcoming and supportive community. *URL: https://www.microdosingforhealing.com/*

MICRODOSING INSTITUTE: a global education, community, and research platform that builds vital connections in society and brings together ancestral wisdom with modern science to allow for safe, conscious, and effective microdosing with psychedelics. *URL: https://microdosinginstitute.com/*

MINDBLOOM: a for-profit mental health and well-being company on a mission to help people expand their human potential. Its goal is bringing clinicians, technologists, and researchers together to increase access to science-backed psychedelic medicine treatments, focused primarily on increasing access to effective science-backed treatments for anxiety and depression, starting with guided ketamine therapy. *URL: https://www.mindbloom.com/*

MULTIDISCIPLINARY ASSOCIATION FOR PSYCHEDELIC STUDIES (MAPS): one of the best-known organizations leading the charge of psychedelics into therapeutic medicines. It is a nonprofit research and educational organization working to raise awareness and understanding of psychedelic substances. *URL: https://maps.org/*

NATIONAL PSYCHEDELICS ASSOCIATION: a nonprofit creating products, services, and infrastructure essential to overcome challenges so that non-prescription psychedelic-assisted care can expand safely and consistently across the US. Has a mission of ensuring everyone in the U.S. can and will get the support they need accessing psychedelic-assisted therapy. *URL: https://www.yournpa.org/*

PEOPLE OF COLOR PSYCHEDELIC COLLECTIVE: a nonprofit that supports healing and justice in communities of color through knowledge and expertise of psychedelics. The organization is committed to a psychedelic revolution that increases accessibility, as well as financial and technical infrastructure, to communities of color while reducing harm and dangers stemming from lack of diversity. *URL: https://www.pocpc.org/*

PLANT MEDICINE COALITION: a nonprofit with a mission to create, protect, and promote safe, equitable access to natural and synthetic psychedelic plant medicines through local and national advocacy. *URL: https://www.plantmedicinefoundation.org/*

PLANT MEDICINE HEALING ALLIANCE: A nonprofit with a mission to decriminalize fungi and plant medicines for home growing, group healing, and ceremonial and religious purposes… promoting sustainable sourcing and honoring, in mutual reciprocity of care, the human, plant, and animal ecologies where the medicines grow. *URL: https://plantmedicinehealing.org/*

PSYCHABLE: created to be a community, connecting people who are exploring the power of psychedelic-assisted therapy with practitioners who can support them. As the legal landscape continues to shift, it wants to simplify the process of finding experienced professionals offering legal healing modalities (i.e. ketamine-assisted therapy, somatic healing, and breathwork) along with those that can help patients with their pre- and post-psychedelic experiences. *URL: https:// psychable.com/*

PSYCHE: a digital magazine from Aeon that illuminates the human condition through psychology, philosophy, and the arts, disseminating knowledge from a wide range of expert perspectives. Psychology and philosophy are key, but it also draws on history, anthropology, and other disciplines. *URL: https://psyche.co/*

THE PSYCHEDELIC: is "a treasure box filled with powerful insights, deep research, and critical news all about the world of entheogens and psychedelics." Includes detailed information on Ayahuasca, DMT, kratom, MDMA, mescaline, and psilocybin. *URL: https://thepsychedelic.com/*

PSYCHEDELIC ACCESS DIRECTORY: a directory for the BIPOC community, where users can easily search its Queer or BIPOC Psychedelic Provider, finding a trusted network of top-rated psychotherapists, physicians, nurses, and community healers. *URL: http://www.psychedelicaccessdirectory.com/*

PSYCHEDELIC EXPERIENCE: a comprehensive online resource for information surrounding psychedelic substances. Its mission is to support and facilitate global healing and personal growth through safe, responsible, and legal use of plant medicines and psychedelic-assisted treatments. *URL: https://www.psychedelicexperience.net/*

PSYCHEDELIC FRONTIER: dedicated to empowering individuals to make safe and intelligent decisions regarding their own consciousness, with information designed with the purpose of education and harm reduction. It encourages the responsible exploration of non-ordinary mental states, including the use of psychedelics by qualified persons in safe and legal settings. *URL: http://psychedelicfrontier.com/*

PSYCHEDELIC INSIGHTS: A for-profit organization with a mission to help people enhance personal growth and development through a well-prepared safe set and setting for guided psychedelic experiences, focused on psilocybin truffles in the Netherlands. It focuses on innovating personal transformation to accelerate the tipping point of human consciousness. *URL: https://psychedelicinsights.com/*

PSYCHEDELIC MEDICINE COALITION: a women-led, nonprofit advocacy organization that believes natural psychedelic plant medicines and their synthetic relatives hold vast potential as tools for improving the health and wellness of individuals and their communities. *URL: https://psychedelicmedicinecoalition.org/*

PSYCHEDELIC NEWS WIRE (PNW): is a specialized content distribution company that (1) aggregates and distributes news and information on the latest developments in all aspects and advances of psychedelics and their use. PNW is committed to delivering improved visibility and brand recognition to companies operating in the emerging markets of psychedelics. *URL: https://www.psychedelicnewswire.com/*

PSYCHEDELIC PASSAGE: is a for-profit organization comprising a network of U.S.-based psychedelic guides & tripsitters who facilitate in-person ceremonial psychedelic experiences with an emphasis on harm reduction. "We foster transformational journeys through the exploration of consciousness, which we believe to be a fundamental human right." *URL: https://www.psychedelicpassage.com/*

PSYCHEDELIC SCIENCE REVIEW: discusses scientific research and knowledge about psychedelics, from chemistry to psychology – where science writers break down complex topics, offering context and connecting important concepts in the literature to familiar examples. It also offers background information about psychedelic compounds, an ever-changing history of events surrounding psychedelics, and the organizations and people involved in progressing the field. *URL: https://psychedelicreview.com/*

PSYCHEDELIC SISTERHOOD: BIPOC-founded, womxn-led community dedicated to creating safe spaces for womxn and gender non-conforming persons to rediscover their relationship to the cosmos and the divine feminine through altered states. It encourages examining "alternative healing methods in melting away normative labels so that we can naturally traverse our true selves." *URL: https://www.thepsychedelicsisterhood.com/*

PSYCHEDELIC SOCIETIES: catalogs the more than 100 psychedelic societies, meetups, and groups around the world for people seeking a local and reliable source of information about psychedelics; these groups sponsor book clubs, group discussions, documentary viewings, workshops, visiting speakers, and other events. From The Psychedelic. *URL: https://thepsychedelic.com/psychedelic-societies/*

PSYCHEDELIC SPOTLIGHT: its mission is to help people obtain a reliable source for the latest stories in the emerging psychedelics industry, covering breakthrough discoveries, investor news, and cultural reform. *URL: https://psychedelicspotlight.com/*

PSYCHEDELIC SUPPORT: designed as a platform to accelerate personal and global transformation by advancing responsible psychedelic-assisted therapy and is a leading education and therapeutic platform – advocating for mental health and well-being worldwide. *URL: https://psychedelic.support/*

PSYCHEDELIC TIMES: its mission is to share the latest news, research, and happenings around the study of psychedelics as tools of healing, recovery, and therapy. Focused on the incredible potential that psychoactive substances such as cannabis, Ayahuasca, MDMA, LSD, iboga, psilocybin, and DMT present to humanity. *URL: https://psychedelictimes.com/*

PSYCHEDELICS DAILY: has as its mission to be the voice for the psychedelic community, to present well-researched, high-quality material and advice on the responsible and effective use of psychedelics for living happier and healthier lives. Also, to influence public opinion sufficiently through education and raising awareness to legalize the responsible use of psychedelic drugs by adults. *URL: https://www.psychedelicsdaily.com/*

PSYCHEDELICS TODAY: is dedicated to exploring and discussing the important academic/scientific and other research in the field of psychedelics, with a particular interest in how psychedelics and other non-ordinary states of consciousness relate to the human potential, as well as the healing potential that they can foster. *URL: https://psychedelicstoday.com/*

REALITY SANDWICH: is a free public education platform with more than 5,000 pieces of content, serving up a full spread of psychedelic information, including a plethora of research, news, and culture to enhance your knowledge of psychedelics, as well as user guides and interviews with experts in the field of psychedelic research. *URL: https://realitysandwich.com/*

ROLLSAFE.ORG: an educational website about MDMA, with numerous articles and useful information on safe practices with MDMA. *URL: https://rollsafe.org/*

SABE JOURNEYS: a Public Benefit Corporation and veteran-owned business, helping to expand veteran access to psychedelic healing through focused retreats and the nonprofit organizations Heroic Hearts Project and the H.O.P.E Project. These cooperative missions provide hope and healing from PTSD, TBI, trauma, depression, and more, to our nation's veterans and military families. *URL: https://sabejourneys.org/*

SISTERS IN PSYCHEDELICS: with a mission to create a community and a platform that empowers people to elevate the divine feminine and other underrepresented voices in the evolution of the psychedelic ecosystem... offering engagement, inspiration, acceptance, and healing – to all. *URL: https://sistersin-psychedelics.org/*

SOCIEDELIC: is a nonprofit community dedicated to promoting knowledge and responsible use of psychedelic compounds and provides journalism on natural therapies and medicines to enhance the mind, body, and spirit. It shares the latest news, research, and happenings around the study of psychedelics as tools of healing, recovery, and therapy. *URL: https://www.sociedelic.com/*

SPORE (SOCIETY FOR PSYCHEDELIC OUTREACH, REFORM, EDUCATION): is a nonprofit with a mission as a community organizing and educational media platform – promoting community health and wealth, equity and justice, and responsible stewardship with psychedelics. *URL: https://www.thespore.org/*

THE THIRD WAVE: has as a mission to share trusted, research-based content that helps people feel safe, supported, and empowered as they follow their path toward personal transformation. Its vision is to help co-create a global movement that embraces psychedelic use to heal ourselves and our world, offering a cohesive platform that meets individual needs, offers guided support, enables integrated experiences, and fosters meaningful connections across our global ecosystem. *URL: https://thethirdwave.co/*

TRIPPYWIKI: has as a mission to help people find the right psychedelics and use them safely and effectively, helping society integrate psychedelics. Offers guides on many psychedelic medicines, including LSD, DMT, ketamine, peyote, Ibogaine, MDMA, psilocybin, 5-MeO DMT, Ayahuasca, cannabis, and many more. *URL: https://trippywiki.com/*

TRIPSAFE.ORG: an educational website about psychedelics, with a main focus on LSD and Psilocybin/Magic Mushrooms, as well as others. *URL: https://tripsafe.org/*

TRIPSITTER: an educational resource exploring the safe and responsible use of psychedelics, serving as a guide and offering support in preparation for a psychedelic journey. Includes well-researched content to help people understand how psychedelics work and how to use them safely for the purpose of personal growth and development. *URL: https://tripsitter.com/*

TRIPSITTERS: has as its mission to manage a loving, supportive community of psychonauts and facilitators. Providing resources, education, and guidance for every step of the healing journey. Its vision is a healthy and happy world where everyone has safe access to psychedelic medicines. *URL: https://www.tripsitters.org/*

TRUFFLE REPORT: is dedicated to bringing readers the best of the burgeoning psychedelic space through high-quality content and original storytelling… with a goal of driving the mainstreaming of psychedelics across legal, business, cultural, and medical and scientific channels. *URL: https://truffle.report/*

VETERANS OF WAR: nonprofit that connects teams of veterans to psychedelic-assisted guided group therapy designed to heal the scars of war in community. *URL: https://www.veteransofwar.org/*

VETS (VETERANS EXPLORING TREATMENT SOLUTIONS): a nonprofit with a mission to end the veteran suicide epidemic by providing resources, research, and advocacy for U.S. military veterans seeking psychedelic-assisted therapies for traumatic brain injury (TBI), post-traumatic stress disorder (PTSD), addition, and other health conditions. *URL: https://vetsolutions.org/*

WOMEN ON PSYCHEDELICS (WOOP): is an educational platform and a global community of female psychedelic enthusiasts and professionals who believe in the transformative potential of psychedelics… and to the end of the stigmatization around women's mental health and women's drug use. *URL: https://www.womenonpsychedelics.org/*

ZENDO PROJECT: a nonprofit organization committed to peer support services, providing professional comprehensive harm reduction education and support for communities to help inform and transform difficult (bad, challenging) psychedelic experiences into opportunities for learning and growth. *URL: https://zendoproject.org/*

....

PSYCHEDELIC PODCASTS

ADVENTURES THROUGH THE MIND: Hosted by James. W. Jesso, this podcast covers numerous topics – all grounded in psychedelics and the mind. Topics range from spirituality, mental health, and emotional maturity; to love, relationships and sexuality; to history, philosophy, and neuroscience. *URL: https://www.jameswjesso.com/podcast/*

AYAHUASCA TALKS: Hosted by Rebecca Hayden, an Ayahuasca integration coach and mental health advocate, focuses on Ayahuasca integration, with discussion about how the medicine changes our minds, hearts, lives – and the world around us. *URL: https://rebeccahayden.com/Ayahuasca-talks-podcast/*

CELEBRATING WOMEN IN PSYCHEDELICS: Hosted by Sonia Stringer, a passionate advocate for psychedelic-assisted therapy who has devoted her entire career to studying traditional and innovative approaches to psychology and personal transformation. Learn how women are shaping the emerging psychedelic landscape – and connect with women involved in psychedelics around the world. *URL: https://www.celebrating-women-in-psychedelics.com/*

ENTHEOGEN: Hosted by the trio of Joe, Brad, and Kevin, this podcast covers psychedelics and related tools used in therapeutic, medicinal, sacramental, and recreational contexts. *URL: https://entheogenshow.com/*

THE ENTHEOGENIC EVOLUTION: Hosted by Martin W. Ball, features visionaries pioneering the cutting-edge of awakening in psychedelic science, modern shamanism, and visionary culture, with discussions of the nondual and unitary nature of being as revealed by conscious entheogenic energetic awakening as well as broad topics in psychedelics, therapy, philosophy, science, and culture. *URL: https://www.podomatic.com/podcasts/entheogenic/*

HAMILTON MORRIS PODCAST: Hosted by none other than Hamilton Morris, the host of the wonderful Vice show, *Hamilton's Pharmacopeia*, and featuring topics on all areas of psychedelics – including talks with legends in the field, self-experiments with little-known psychedelics, more. *URL: https://hamilton-morris.buzzsprout.com/*

LET'S TALK PLANT MEDICINE: Hosted by Dr. Lara Ohonba, a clinical pharmacist certified in medical cannabis, this podcast covers alternative ways to improve your health and well-being – using the healing power of medicinal herbs such as cannabinoids, psychedelics, and conventional therapy. *URL: https://wci-health.com/podcast/*

MAPS PODCAST: Hosted by Zach Leary, this production from the Multidisciplinary Association for Psychedelic Studies is designed to inspire and ignite your imagination into the world of psychedelic research and culture. Includes unique information sourced from talks, presentations, and panels that have taken place at past *Psychedelic Science* conferences and other unique events. *URL: https://maps.org/news/maps-podcast/*

MICRODOSING THE PODCAST: DEDICATED TO YOUR HEALTH AND WELLNESS JOURNEY: Hosted by Functional Health and Wellness Coach D. Michael Brooks candidly discusses his extensive use of microdosing psychedelic medicine to break his sugar addiction, advance his weight loss journey, and drastically improve his mood and mindfulness. His overall goal is to provide education and offer insights that may be valuable as you decide on an alternative to traditional Western medicine. *URL: https://microdosingthepodcast.com/*

MIKEADELIC: Hosted by Mike Brancatelli, this podcast explores big ideas through a psychedelic point of view with a focus on cognitive liberty. Mike's mission is to create a space for inspiring and unconventional conversations that provoke interesting and unique explorations of deep thoughts and ideas. *URL: https://mikedelic.libsyn.com/*

MINORITY TRIP REPORT: a podcast for under-represented views and life journeys with mental health, psychedelics, and consciousness. Hosted by Raad, a Bangladeshi-Canadian entrepreneur at the trifecta of consciousness, culture, and capital. *URL: https://www.minoritytrip.com/*

PLUS THREE: this podcast takes a deep dive into the world of drugs, from local decriminalization and emerging psychedelic corporations to leftist politics and mass incarceration. Each week the team and guests attempt to make sense of the complex connections between drugs, science, capitalism, policy, and culture. *https://www.psymposia.com/podcasts/plusthree/*

THE PSYCHEDELIC CHRISTIAN PODCAST: Hosted by Clint Kyles, this podcast provides a platform for Christians to share their thoughts and experiences concerning psychedelics with the broader Christian community. The podcast is a space for Christians to learn more about this topic, by witnessing the thoughts, opinions, and experiences of their peers – to supplement the faith community with enough sound information to make practical judgments on this phenomenon. *URL: http://thepsychedelicchristianpodcast.com/*

THE PSYCHEDELIC LEADERSHIP PODCAST: Hosted by Laura Dawn, and with a focus on conversations about how we can learn to embody heart-centered leadership so we can influence real change and create a more beautiful world – exploring the intersection between psychedelics and sacred plant medicines, neuroscience and consciousness, creativity and resilience, business and entrepreneurship, meaning and purpose. *URL: https://lauradawn.co/psychedelic-leadership-podcast/*

PSYCHEDELIC MEDICINE PODCAST: Hosted by Dr. Lynn Marie Morski, this podcast focuses on demystifying and destigmatizing plant medicines through education – of both the medical establishment and others who could potentially benefit from these medicines. *URL: https://www.plantmedicine.org/podcast/*

PSYCHEDELIC PASSAGE PODCAST: Hosted by professional psychedelic guides and facilitators Nicholas Levich and Jimmy Nguyen, the focus of this podcast is providing tips and best practices, as well as answering common questions about safely using psychedelics for meaningful change. *URL: https://www.psychedelicpassage.com/podcasts/*

THE PSYCHEDELIC PSYCHOLOGIST: Hosted by integration expert Dr. Ryan Westrum, this conversational-style podcast includes clients and other guests who use talk therapy to integrate psychedelic experiences for healing and personal transformation. *URL: https://podbay.fm/p/the-psychedelic-psychologist/*

PSYCHEDELIC RADIO: this podcast aims to illuminate and destigmatize the use of psychedelic medicines and provide real insight into the paradigm shift that is forming around how mental health is treated. Charles Patti and Christina Thomas discuss how psychedelic medicine is being used to treat a myriad of mental health issues. *URL: https://cannabisradio.com/audio/8003/*

PSYCHEDELIC SALON: Hosted by Lorenzo Hagerty, with a focus on the use and benefits of psychoactive plants and chemicals, both in their natural settings and in medical research. More than 650+ episodes. *URL: https://psychedelicsalon.com/podcasts/*

PSYCHEDELIC SPOTLIGHT PODCAST: covers the latest stories in the emerging psychedelics industry, including breakthrough discoveries, investor news, and cultural reform, to develop a powerful and intuitive network for collaboration with industry leaders, researchers, and investors who are transcending the way the world regards what is possible in mental health, the mind and human consciousness. *URL: https://psychedelicspotlight.com/psychedelic-community/podcast/*

PSYCHEDELIC THERAPY FRONTIERS: Hosted by Dr. Steve Thayer and Dr. Reid Robison, this podcast explores the frontiers of psychedelic medicine and what it takes to cultivate a healthy mind, body, and spirit, as well as discussing the science, practice, and art of psychedelic healing. *URL: https://www.psychedelictherapyfrontiers.com/*

THE PSYCHEDELIC THERAPY PODCAST: Hosted by Eamon Armstrong, this podcast focuses on conversations with leaders in the psychedelic community – and is specifically designed for therapists, healers, retreat leaders, and passionate enthusiasts. *URL: https://www.mayahealth.com/podcast/*

PSYCHEDELIC TIMES PODCAST: Hosted by Wesley Thoricatha, the focus is on sharing the latest news, research, and happenings around the study of psychedelics as tools of healing, recovery, and therapy. *URL: https://psychedelictimes.com/category/podcasts/*

PSYCHEDELICS TODAY: Hosted by Joe Moore and Kyle Buller, this podcast focuses on important academic and other research in the field of psychedelics. It discusses how psychedelics relate to human potential and healing. *URL: https://psychedelicstoday.com/podcast/*

THE THIRD WAVE: Hosted by Paul Austin, this podcast explores the many minds of the emerging psychedelic renaissance. Through conversations with thought leaders across various disciplines, it explores how psychedelics, when used with intention and responsibility, catalyze transformation on both an individual and collective level. *URL: https://thethirdwave.co/podcast/*

TRUELIFE: Hosted by the affable George Monty, this podcast takes a deep dive into the depths of the unconscious mind. Psychology, philosophy, psychedelic research and social engineering are but a few of the topics investigated. Tactical empathy, purple dawn theory, beautiful beaches, and book reviews. *URL: https:// podcasts.google.com/search/TrueLife/*

THE VINE: An insightful look into the world of plant medicine. Exploring the changing landscape around cannabis and psychedelics, and ending the stigma through educational discussions. From the Plant Media Project and hosted by the co-founders Gina Vensel and Elizabeth Sheldon. *URL: https://www.plantmediaproject.com/blog/*

WORTH THE FIGHT PODCAST: If you're curious about psychedelic medicines, flow states, and how our deepest traumas just might be our greatest hidden strengths, then check out this podcast hosted by Matt Simpson. Find guests who, through their journey and transformation, tell their stories of hope, healing, and expansion. "With each episode, we activate hearts and minds, reminding ourselves we are all worth the fight." *URL: https://wtfpodcast.org/*

....

PSYCHEDELIC YOUTUBE CHANNELS

BEYOND THE MEDICINE – HOLO THERAPEUTICS: where you can find video content on psychedelics, plant medicines, and entheogens produced by Holo Therapeutics (https://hololife.health/). Find video interviews and stories of healing with people and professionals in the psychedelic community, and professionals who have used psychedelics to expand their worlds. Discover the power of psychedelics to help create real-life changes. *URL: https://www.youtube.com/channel/UCd31EgDc0XuCI1chfxFVjRA/*

HIGH PRIESTESS HEALING: a video channel from healer Jessica Posillico, Reiki Master and certified life coach. Several videos on her channel focus on Ayahuasca – prep, journey, and integration. (Review her story in Chapter 10.) *URL: https://www.youtube.com/channel/UCSieHs4A1Xe19uN80ankzKA/*

APPENDIX 2:

Psychedelic Books and Documentary Movies/Series

This appendix is divided into print and streaming. The first section will cover books and the second section documentaries streaming on various platforms. All of these resources are some of the best for continuing your education into psychedelic medicine and healing through psychedelics.

BOOKS ABOUT PSYCHEDELICS

If you are looking to take a deep dive into psychedelics and psychedelic plant medicines, then this list of 30+ books should keep you busy for some time! Any and all of these books make an excellent addition to your psychedelic library and to your greater understanding of this interesting field.

I have tried to include a broad selection of books, from some basic books on using psychedelics to books that have a specific focus on one or more of these psychedelic medicines.

Ayahuasca Awakening A Guide to Self-Discovery, Self-Mastery and Self-Care: Volume One Self-Discovery and Self-Mastery (1039115241) AND *Ayahuasca Awakening A Guide to Self-Discovery, Self-Mastery and Self-Care: Volume Two Self-Care and the Circle of Wholeness* (1039115276), by Jessica Rochester, D.Div. Find more than 500 pages of detailed, inspirational, and powerful content spread across two volumes; designed as a guidebook for personal and spiritual development.

Psychedelic Wisdom: The Astonishing Rewards of Mind-Altering Substances, by Richard Louis Miller, Ph.D. (with chapter contributions from many other experts). 1644115433. A discussion of how scientists, doctors, therapists, and teachers have applied their entheogenic experiences in their professions, leading to therapeutic advancements, scientific discoveries, and healing for thousands.

The Psychedelic Explorer's Guide: Safe, Therapeutic, and Sacred Journeys, by James Fadiman, Ph.D. 1594774021. Reviews the value of psychedelics for healing and self-discovery as well as how LSD has facilitated scientific and technical problem-solving.

How to Change Your Mind: What the New Science of Psychedelics Teaches Us About Consciousness, Dying, Addiction, Depression, and Transcendence, by Michael Pollan. 1594204225. Presents a remarkable history of psychedelics and a compelling portrait of the new generation of scientists fascinated by the implications of these drugs.

Psychedelics For Everyone: A Beginners Guide to these Powerful Medicines for Anxiety, Depression, Addiction, PTSD, and Expanding Consciousness, by Matt Zemon. 979-8986267432. Provides readers with an inspiring foundation for understanding the profound transformational power of psychedelics, including medically reviewed information from experts in the clinical use of psychedelics.

Psychedelic Integration: Psychotherapy for Non-Ordinary States of Consciousness, by Marc Aixalà. 0907791395. traces the evolution of psychedelic-assisted therapy and integration research from the 1960s to the present moment, explains therapeutic techniques, and outlines a clinician's real-world observations on the deep work of healing. The book offers 11 metaphors for understanding integration and concisely explains the seven dimensions of integration, which the author sees as inextricably linked to preparation and the psychedelic session experience.

The Promise of Psychedelics; Science-Based Hope for Better Mental Health, by Dr. Peter Silverstone. 979-8845820686. Introduces scientific advances in our understanding of psychedelics: how they work, what the risks are, and which ones will transform mental health treatment for millions of patients.

The Psilocybin Connection: Psychedelics, the Transformation of Consciousness, and Evolution on the Planet – An Integral Approach, by Jahan Khamsehzadeh, Ph.D. 1623176549. Explores our historical and ancestral relationship to psychedelics, presents new and exciting research, and explores what psilocybin can mean for us today.

Queering Psychedelics: From Oppression to Liberation in Psychedelic Medicine, edited by Alex Belser, Ph.D., Clancy Cavnar, Psy.D., and Beatriz Caiuby Labate, Ph.D. 1957869038. By addressing and dismantling sexist, heteronormative, transphobic, and homophobic forms of oppression in the psychedelic community, this collection features a broad range of perspectives from queer academic researchers, LGBTQIA+ clinicians, and Indigenous and transgender advocates.

Food of the Gods: The Search for the Original Tree of Knowledge: A Radical History of Plants, Drugs, and Human Evolution, by Terrence McKenna. 0553371304. Showcases research on our ancient relationship with chemicals, opens a doorway to the Divine, and perhaps a solution for saving our troubled world. Includes a revisionist look at the historical role of drugs in the East and the West.

Sacred Medicine: A Doctor's Quest to Unravel the Mysteries of Healing, by Lissa Rankin, MD. 1683647424. Follow Dr. Rankin around the world to meet healers gifted and flawed, go on pilgrimage to sacred sites, investigate the science of healing, and learn how to stay safe when seeking a healer.

Sacred Knowledge: Psychedelics and Religious Experiences, by Dr. William A. Richards. 0231174063. A sophisticated account of the effect of psychedelics on biological processes, human consciousness, and revelatory religious experiences. Follows the belief that, if used responsibly and legally, psychedelics have the potential to assuage suffering and constructively affect the quality of human life.

The God Molecule: 5-MeO-DMT and the Spiritual Path to the Divine Light, by Gerardo Ruben Sandoval, MD. 1611250498. A story of the author's attempt to discover/find the most powerful source of healing energy in the natural world, which he finds in the secretions of the Sonoran Desert toad — the most profound healer of all: 5-MeO-DMT, the God molecule.

DMT: The Spirit Molecule: A Doctor's Revolutionary Research into the Biology of Near-Death and Mystical Experiences, by Rick Strassman, MD. 9780892819270. Read the detailed account of Dr. Rick Strassman, who conducted US DEA-approved clinical research from 1990 to 1995 at the University of New Mexico in which he injected 60 volunteers with DMT, one of the most powerful psychedelics known.

Psychedelic Medicine: The Healing Powers of LSD, MDMA, Psilocybin, and Ayahuasca, by Richard Louis Miller, Ph.D. (with chapter contributions from many other experts). 1620556979. Explores the potential of psychedelics as medicine and the intersections of politics, science, and psychedelics.

The Psychedelic Handbook: A Practical Guide to Psilocybin, LSD, Ketamine, MDMA, and Ayahuasca, by Rick Strassman, MD. 1646043812. Learn everything you need to know about psychedelics with this ultimate guide packed with information on popular psychedelic drugs like psilocybin, ketamine, MDMA, DMT, and LSD... plus practical tips for microdosing and how to safely "trip."

Integration Workbook: Planting Seeds for Growth and Change, by Kyle Buller and Joe Moore. 1986544613. Psychedelic experiences can be difficult, confusing, blissful, and life-changing, but knowing what to do next can be overwhelming. This psychedelic integration workbook is designed to help you through your process. This workbook consists of different activities such as meditation prompts, journaling exercises, and goal planning.

Psychedelics and Spirituality: The Sacred Use of LSD, Psilocybin, and MDMA for Human Transformation, edited by Thomas B. Roberts, Ph.D. 1644110229. Reveals how psychedelics can facilitate spiritual development and direct encounters with the sacred. With contributions by Albert Hofmann, Huston Smith, Stanislav Grof, Charles Tart, Alexander "Sasha" Shulgin, Brother David Steindl-Rast, and many others.

Grandmother Ayahuasca: Plant Medicine and the Psychedelic Brain, by Christian Funder. 1644112353. An exploration of the history, shamanic use, psychoactive effects, current scientific studies, and therapeutic potential of Ayahuasca.

The Entheological Paradigm: Essays on the DMT and 5-MeO-DMT Experience and the Meaning of it All, by Martin W. Ball, Ph.D. 979-8592426919. Leading entheogenic advocate presents a naturalistic, rational, and objective view on the nature of reality as seen through the lenses of DMT and 5-MeO-DMT when appreciated from a radical nondual perspective.

Tripping: An Anthology of True-Life Psychedelic Adventures, edited by Charles Hayes. 0140195742. Includes 50 stories about unforgettable psychedelic experiences from an international array of subjects representing all walks of life, as well as supplemental essays about psychedelics.

The Doors of Perception and Heaven and Hell, by Aldous Huxley. 0061729078. Two of the most profound essays are included in this one volume... exploring the mind's remote frontiers and the unmapped areas of human consciousness.

The Joyous Cosmology: Adventures in the Chemistry of Consciousness, by Alan W. Watts. 9781608682041. Examines how the consciousness-changing drugs LSD, mescaline, and psilocybin can facilitate for people who are looking for understanding and reflection.

Breaking Open the Head: A Psychedelic Journey into the Heart of Contemporary Shamanism, by Daniel Pinchbeck. 0767907434. Explores the author's personal journeys and experiences with various plant substances such as iboga and Ayahuasca, along with his quest for knowledge about shamanism.

Worth The Fight: Acting for a Better World, A Guide to Spirituality, Psyche-delic Medicines and Overcoming Trauma, by Matthew Simpson. 1796938327. A book that provides a hopeful look at how psychedelics, meditation, and flow might impact a world starved of love. The book calls for a love revolution that is fueled by forgiveness, compassion, kindness and selfless service to others.

Plants of the Gods: Their Sacred, Healing, and Hallucinogenic Pow-ers, by Richard Evans Schultes, Albert Hofmann, and Christian Ratsch. 0892819790. Three titans of the field provide insights and depths in this revised version. Explores the uses of hallucinogenic plants in shamanic rituals throughout the world.

LSD: Doorway to the Numinous: The Groundbreaking Psychedelic Research into Realms of the Human Unconscious, by Stanislav Grof, MD. 1594772827. From one of the leading LSD researchers in the world, this book describes the pharmacology of the LSD reaction and goes deeply into reporting and catego-rizing the multi-level and transpersonal aspects of it.

Listening to Ayahuasca: New Hope for Depression, Addiction, PTSD, and Anxiety, by Rachel Harris, Ph.D. 1608684024. The author shares her original research (the largest study of Ayahuasca use in North America) into its effects on depression, anxiety, and PTSD, along with her own personal experiences.

Iboga The Root of All Healing, by Daniel Brett. 1838446214. For those ad-dicted to harmful substances, iboga, and its alkaloid – Ibogaine, represents a po-tent means of interrupting addictions, particularly to opioid-based compounds. However, like iboga itself, this book is not solely for the benefit of addicts, but for people seeking healing and transformation.

A Dose of Hope: A Story of MDMA-Assisted Psychotherapy, by Dan Engle, MD, and Alex Young. 1544521022. A groundbreaking, informative, and easy-to-read book that discusses MDMA treatment through the eyes of a fictional patient so you can see how it works without ever setting foot in a doctor's office. Follow in-depth conversations between doctor and patient, learn about the his-tory of MDMA-assisted therapy, and understand how and why it helps.

Magic Mushroom Explorer: Psilocybin and the Awakening Earth, by Simon G. Powell. 162055366X. A visionary guide to safely using psilocybin mush-rooms to tap into the wisdom of nature and reconnect humanity to the bio-sphere. It explores the ecopsychological effects of wild psychedelic mushrooms, including enhanced biophilia, expanded awareness, eco-shamanic encounters, and access to the ancient wisdom that binds all life on Earth.

Your Brain on Psychedelics: How do Psychedelics Work? Pharmacology and Neuroscience of Psilocybin, DMT, LSD, MDMA, Mescaline, by Genis Ona. 8418943343. With this guide you will learn the keys to the effects of psychedelics, which are capable of producing significant changes in the processes of perception, thought and consciousness.

The Beginners Introductory Guide to DMT - Psychedelics and The Dimethyltryptamine Molecule, by Alex Gibbons. 1095584812. Full of fascinating stories. Explore the effects of DMT including the risks and benefits of taking it in the modern world. Educate yourself and learn the history of this psychedelic compound before you decide to go further.

The Psychedelics Integration Handbook, by Ryan Westrum, Ph.D., and Jay Dufrechou, Ph.D. 173387660X. Designed to bring psychedelic experiences into the flow of your life and maximize their potential for helping you create the life you want to live. This is not a book with black and white answers but an offering to individual people who want to explore all the possibilities for being alive and seeking wholeness.

....

AND FOR THOSE CONSIDERING MICRODOSING RATHER THAN MACRODOSING, CHECK OUT...

Microdosing Psychedelics: A Practical Guide to Upgrade Your Life, by Paul Austin. 1980670919. A comprehensive guide to all the necessary information on the practice of microdosing – including protocols, benefits, drawbacks, and sourcing. Oriented toward anyone interested in microdosing to improve their general well-being.

The Microdosing Guidebook: A Step-by-Step Manual to Improve Your Physical and Mental Health through Psychedelic Medicine, by C. J. Spotswood, PMHNP. 1646043103. Learn about the history, research, and helpful effects of microdosing psychedelic medicines like psilocybin, LSD, ecstasy, and more with this combination manual and workbook.

Integrate: 3 Month Microdosing Guide, by Kristin Taylor. 1387719580. This guide/journal allows an intuitive way to process the learning, lessons and creativity that comes along with the microdosing journey. The medicine is the doorway, integration is the path.

The Science of Microdosing Psychedelics, by Torsten Passie, MD. 099280888X. A carefully researched and scientifically presented book that provides an objective and clear perspective on microdosing LSD and other psychedelics, covering key areas such as history, tolerance, toxicity, and placebo.

The Complete Guide to Microdosing Psilocybin Mushrooms | Guidebook & Journal: An All-Inclusive Beginners Guide to Microdosing Psilocybin Mushrooms & a Microdosing Journal, by Alan Alpert. 979-8845820686. An all-inclusive beginners guide to microdosing psilocybin mushrooms – along with a detailed microdosing journal for integration.

....

DOCUMENTARIES ABOUT PSYCHEDELICS

If you are looking to explore and enhance your knowledge of plant medicines and psychedelics (including tetrahydrocannabinol-THC from cannabis, psilocybin, Ayahuasca, mescaline, Ibogaine, bufotenine, MDMA, LSD, ketamine, and others), then this list of documentary films and series is for you.

While you will find many of the same experts and researchers discussing psychedelics in these documentaries, the perspective is often different... and some focus on just one psychedelic medicine, while others cover even some very obscure psychedelics.

Most of these documentaries look at the progress in the research (now finally being renewed after almost five decades of being banned) of psychedelics for dealing with such a wide variety of mental and health issues, including addiction, depression, anxiety, OCD, post-traumatic stress, Alzheimer's disease, and more.

Most of these documentaries are streaming on the major platforms (Netflix, Hulu, Amazon, YouTube) ... and more are coming!

....

MOVIES

Ayahuasca: Vine of the Soul (2010). A documentary set in the heart of the Amazon, a naturopathic doctor and an accountant experience life-altering epiphanies when they drink the psychoactive brew Ayahuasca, the 'Vine of the Soul.'

AYA: Awakenings (2013). This documentary is adapted from a book by Taz Razam titled *Aya: A Shamanic Odyssey.* It explores the modern business of Westerners traveling to the Amazon and Ayahuasca shamanism as it relates to "spiritual tourism" and how this industry clashes with the traditional view of shamanism.

Dirty Pictures (2010). Examines the amazing work and life of Dr. Alexander "Sasha" Shulgin and takes viewers inside his Northern California home where he lived with his wife of 40 years. (He and his wife are now both dead.) The movie also covers some of the spiritual aspects of psychedelics as well as the psychotherapy aspects of MDMA and current ongoing research in the medical field.

Dosed (2019). directed by Tyler Chandler, centers around the filmmaker's friend, who is a drug addict seeking recovery by using psychedelics – starting with a low dose of psilocybin before moving to a therapeutic dose for relief. Eventually, the narrator turns to a retreat where she tries iboga. The filmmakers have recently filmed a follow up: *Dosed2.*

DMT: The Spirit Module (2010). Based on the book by Dr. Rick Strassman (the first doctor to undertake human research with psychedelic, hallucinogenic, or entheogenic substances), with Joe Rogan as narrator, this documentary investigates the mystery of dimethyltryptamine (DMT), a molecule found in nearly every living organism – and considered the most potent psychedelic on Earth.

Fantastic Fungi (2019). A consciousness-shifting documentary about the mycelium network that takes us on an immersive journey through time and scale into the magical earth beneath our feet, an underground network that can heal and save our planet.

From Shock to Awe (2018). An intimate and raw look at the transformational journey of two combat veterans suffering from severe trauma as they abandon pharmaceuticals to seek relief through the mind-expanding world of psychedelics.

Inside LSD (2009). From National Geographic, this film explores how renewed research in psychedelics is changing lives for patients in clinical trials, as well as researchers; includes interviews with several professionals in the Multidisciplinary Association for Psychedelic Studies (MAPS) as well as a subject in one of the studies.

The Medicine (2020). A documentary that reveals the hidden mysteries of one of nature's most powerful and controversial healing remedies, Ayahuasca. The film explores the science as well as the lore behind the plant and why it is used to heal.

The Nature of Ayahuasca (2019). Exploring the use of Ayahuasca as a holistic medicine, challenging stigmas around its use, and helping people become more conscious and ethical consumers of the plant.

Neurons to Nirvana (2013). Through interviews with the world's foremost researchers, writers, and psychologists, the film explores the history of five powerful psychedelic substances and their previously established medicinal potential. From Canadian filmmaker Oliver Hockenhull.

Psyched Out: Documentary on Psychedelics, Ayahuasca and Plant Medicine (2018). A documentary exploring ancient plant medicines and psychedelics that have been used for thousands of years for healing and spiritual connection – with an attempt to show a different perspective.

Psychedelia: The History and Science of Mystical Experience (2021). A short film that examines the history of psychedelic medicines and their ability to produce mystical experiences – including a look back to the 1960s when psychedelics were considered one of the most promising discoveries in psychology.

Revealing the Mind: The Promise of Psychedelics (2019). A documentary that includes interviews with scientists and psychonauts who are now picking up where research left off 50 years ago when President Nixon made all psychedelics a Schedule 1 Drug, killing all the research being done on healing. Topics include LSD, psilocybin, DMT and other psychedelics to heal—and reveal—the mind.

....

SERIES

Hamilton's Pharmacopeia (2016-2019). From Hamilton Morris, the son of Errol Morris and a true science-geek, a multi-season docuseries that follows Hamilton's travels around the globe exploring the history, science, and social impact of psychoactive substances. Definitely must-see.

Healing Powers of Weed, Psychedelics, & Other Mindful Practices (2018). From documentarian Mareesa Stertz, *a* series of bite-sized episodes on the healing powers of various substances. Wish there were lots more episodes.

How to Change Your Mind (2022). This series, based on the book by Michael Pollan by the same name, explores the history and use of psychedelics, including LSD, psilocybin, MDMA, and mescaline.

Psychedelica (2018-2019). A two-season docuseries that explores the history and use of psychedelic plants as a gateway to expanded consciousness and plant medicine's continued influence on humanity. Lots of great topics covered.

PSYCHEDELIC GLOSSARY

This glossary is not meant to be exhaustive, but to cover all the topics raised in the book – key topics that perhaps need more illumination here.

5-MEO-DMT: a psychedelic medicine of the tryptamine class so powerful that it was named "the God Molecule." It is four to six times more powerful than DMT (the medicine found in Ayahuasca). Naturally, it can be found in a wide variety of trees and shrubs, often alongside DMT and bufotenine (5-HO-DMT), as well as one species of toad. The medicine has also been synthetically produced.

ADDICTION: a chronic dysfunction of the brain system involving a person craving a substance that helps the user escape discomfort and reality (typically from past trauma). The addiction can get even strong with a lack of concern over consequences. Addiction may involve the use of substances such as alcohol, inhalants, opioids, cocaine, and nicotine, or compulsive behaviors such as gambling, sex/cheating, shopping, eating.

ANTIDEPRESSANTS: prescription drugs marketed as relieving the symptoms of depression; designed for short-term use, but many take for decades. Antidepressants are classified into different types depending on their structure and the way that they work, including: monoamine oxidase inhibitors (MAOIs), selective serotonin reuptake inhibitors (SSRIs), serotonin antagonist and reuptake inhibitors (SARIs), serotonin and norepinephrine reuptake inhibitors (SNRIs), and norepinephrine and dopamine reuptake inhibitors (NDRIs)

ANXIETY: while a normal and necessary emotion, it is the most common mental illness diagnosed in the U.S., with approximately 1-in-8 Americans affected by some degree of excessive levels of nervousness, fear, apprehension, and worry – generalized anxiety disorder (GAD). Mild anxiety can be vague and unsettling while severe anxiety can have major impacts on daily living. Anxiolytics are used to treat symptoms of anxiety disorders.

ANXIOLYTICS: prescription drugs used to treat various anxiety disorders and more commonly known as anti-anxiety medications or minor tranquilizers; they are thought to work on key chemical messengers in the brain, helping to decrease abnormal excitability. Some of the more frequently prescribed anxiolytics are benzodiazepines, including: alprazolam (Xanax), chlordiazepoxide (Librium), clonazepam (Klonopin), diazepam (Valium), and lorazepam (Ativan). Note: these drugs are habit-forming and can lead to dependency.

AYAHUASCA: a psychedelic medicine that is known as the "vine of the soul." It is prepared from the combination of the Ayahuasca vine and the leaves of the Chacruna shrub – both of which grow naturally in the Amazon in South America. Also called caapi, yaje, or yage, this DMT-infused tea has been used for healing and community for thousands of years, though traditionally, only the shaman (or healers) drank the tea. Drinking the tea causes altered states of consciousness, including visual hallucinations and altered perceptions of reality.

BAD TRIP: No such thing. See: *challenging trip.*

CANNABIS: a master plant that is worthy of study and medicinal use – one that can even have some psychoactive properties – though most experts do not consider cannabis to be a psychedelic. That said, research is discovering amazing benefits from cannabis, especially in relation to post-traumatic stress, inflammation, anxiety, pain, and sleep. (Other names associated with cannabis include hemp, CBD, marijuana, THC.)

CHALLENGING TRIP: many psychedelic journeys, especially at higher doses, are going to present some intense and challenging memories and images. We used to call these "bad trips" because recreational users (as well as anti-psychedelics propaganda) portrayed these experiences as fearful and dangerous – when in reality, we need to face these images for healing to occur. The more trauma you have experienced, the higher the likelihood of a challenging (but not bad) trip. It's because some journeys can be challenging that many recommend people have support – of a clinician, facilitator, guide, tripsitter, or sober friend.

CONTROLLED SUBSTANCES ACT (CSA): established a federal policy to regulate the manufacturing, distributing, importing/exporting, and use of regulated substances. The CSA was enacted by Congress and signed by President Richard Nixon into law in 1970. The law places all substances that are in some manner regulated under existing federal law into one of five schedules – based upon the substance's supposed medical use, potential for abuse, and safety or dependence liability. All psychedelics (many of which had proven medical benefits before the law went into effect) are currently illegal under the CSA, though new clinical trials may finally result in reclassification of several psychedelic medicines.

DEFAULT MODE NETWORK (DMN): is a system of connected brain areas that show increased activity when a person is not focused on what is happening around them. When the brain is directed toward a task or goal, the default network deactivates. "Default mode" was first used by Dr. Marcus Raichle in 2001 to describe resting brain function. It's been shown that psychedelics such as LSD, psilocybin, Ayahuasca, and others operate to significantly reduce activity in the brain's default mode network (DMN). This reduction in DMN activity functions as a kind of *rebooting* of the brain, and is thought to be linked to one of the most enduring therapeutic effects of psychedelic substances.

DEPRESSION: also called major depressive disorder or clinical depression, it is a mood disorder that causes a persistent feeling of sadness and loss of interest – affecting how people feel, think, and behave – and which can lead to a variety of emotional and physical problems. New research is now questioning several of the major assumptions made about depression and the brain. Depression has traditionally been treated with prescription medications (antidepressants), talk-therapy (psychotherapy), or a combination of the two. Psychedelic medicines (particularly psilocybin and MDMA) are being studied for possible FDA approval for treating depression and so-called treatment-resistant depression.

DMT: N,N-Dimethyltryptamine is a psychedelic chemical that occurs naturally in many plants and animals, including human beings, and which is both a derivative and a structural analog of tryptamine. As DMT, this medicine is ingested in crystal form, smoked it in a pipe or bong, as well as vaporized – producing a powerful, but short-lasting hallucinogenic state, considered to be one of the most intense psychedelic experiences in existence. DMT is also the active hallucinogenic compound in Ayahuasca.

EGO DEATH/DISSOLUTION: is a "complete loss of subjective self-identity" that occurs during higher-dosed psychedelic medicine journeys; it is the temporary loss of one's sense of self. The feeling is usually captured by statements like "I felt at one with the universe" or "I lost all sense of myself." Ego dissolution can help people incorporate less ego and more soul into their daily lives – providing better introspection and disrupting negative patterns of behavior. However, in some cases, instead of the ego shrinking (in relation to the immensity of the universe), the ego expands (feeding the shadow self).

ENTHEOGEN: a psychoactive, hallucinogenic substance or preparation (such as psilocybin, Ibogaine, or Ayahuasca) that results in transcendental experiences – especially when derived from plants or fungi and used in religious, spiritual, or ritualistic contexts. There now exist many synthetic drugs with similar psychoactive properties, many of which are derived from these plants. Chemist and botanical researcher Jonathan Ott is credited with coining the term, which literally means "God within us," in 1979. Often used interchangeably with hallucinogens, psychedelics, psychotomimetics.

FACILITATOR/GUIDE: is a professional with specific training and experience to help guide a psychedelic journey. A facilitator/guide helps provide direction, safety (harm reduction), and security when working with psychedelic or altered states of consciousness. They provide a safe and secure "container" for the psychedelic experience – the structure and support to help focus on your journey – equipped and prepared to help unlock more powerful experiences or deeper truths, ensuring a safe and powerful experience.

FOUR PILLARS OF SAFE PSYCHEDELIC USE: many experts recommend, especially for those first experiencing psychedelic medicines outside of clinical settings, these four elements be in place before starting any psychedelic journey. These pillars include: set (mindset), setting (location), sitter, and substance. One must have the proper intentions/mindset, in a comfortable and safe environment, being watched over by a sitter (or guide or facilitator), with knowledge of the purity and dose of the medicine to be consumed.

HALLUCINOGENS: a diverse group of drugs that alter a person's awareness of their surroundings as well as their own thoughts and feelings. They are commonly split into two categories: classic hallucinogens (such as LSD) and dissociative drugs (such as ketamine). Hallucinogens can be naturally extracted from plants or fungi (such as with Ayahuasca) or can be purely synthetic, produced chemically. Hallucinogens work at least partially by temporarily disrupting communication between chemical systems throughout the brain and spinal cord.

HEROIC DOSE: first coined by guru Terence Mckenna (an American ethnobotanist and mystic) in reference to consuming 5 grams of dry psilocybin mushrooms in a specific, isolated setting. However, as psychedelic medicines have become more popular, the term references a large dose across all the medicines – a dose large enough to result in a powerful and life-changing experience, including ego dissolution. It's best to work with a clinician, coach, guide to get the best dosing for your situation.

IBOGAINE: a naturally occurring psychoactive substance used for medicinal and ritual purposes in African spiritual traditions of the Bwiti religion in Gabon. It was first promoted as having anti-addictive properties in 1962 by Howard Lotsof, who was a heroin addict himself. In France, it was marketed as Lambarene and used as a stimulant. The U.S. Central Intelligence Agency (CIA) also studied the effects of Ibogaine in the 1950s. It's the most gnarly psychedelic and is primarily used in treating addiction to opiates and other highly-addictive drugs, though it is also becoming more common as a tool for personal transformation and spiritual development.

ICAROS: Icaro means "song," or more specifically, a sacred medicine song – typically used in traditional Ayahuasca ceremonies. Icaros are specific to certain regions and teachers/healers, and are sung in different languages. Icaros are seen as powerful tools that help with healing, calling on the healing properties of the plants.

INTEGRATION: tools used to help figure out how to incorporate the lessons learned from a psychedelic journey into your life... figure out how to heal from any previously unknown traumas, figure out what all the images you saw mean, what the whole experience means. People can do most of the integrating by themselves, contemplating all that they discovered in their journey; or, people can integrate with others – including hiring an integration coach. Integration is an ongoing process – and some would say a lifelong process. Learn more in Chapter 3.

INTENTION: a clear statement of your goals or motivations for your psychedelic journey. Intentions help keep us focused on that goal, even if/when a journey gets challenging. Intentions can be fairly open and general, such as "show me what part of me needs healing." But intentions can also be very specific, such as "help me heal from my childhood sexual abuse" or "Help me break my addiction to alcohol." Why bother with an intention, especially if the medicine will show you what it wants to show you? When you are intentional about something, you're more focused, thoughtful, and in the here-and-now.

JOURNEY: consuming a psychedelic medicine produces a temporary change in our mental and physical states, releasing us from old and limiting patterns of self-identification, and propelling us onward into odd and mystical experiences – what's called a journey (and in hippie lingo, a trip). Each medicine has different aspects to a journey, including intensity and duration length, so conduct your research and know exactly what to expect on your journey – given the medicine and the dosage you plan to consume.

KETAMINE: is a NMDA-based dissociative (which works by blocking NMDA receptors), and dates back to 1962 when it was first synthesized by American scientist Calvin Stevens at the Parke Davis Laboratories; it's a medication primarily used for induction and maintenance of anesthesia. It induces dissociative anesthesia, a trance-like state providing pain relief, sedation, and amnesia – and is considered a hallucinogen – but not a classic psychedelic (such as LSD, psilocybin, mescaline, DMT).

LEMON TEK TEA: a method of consuming magic mushrooms that can shorten the duration of a journey and decrease nausea, but can also make the whole experience more intense. It involves steeping dried mushrooms in lemon or lime juice before consumption – essentially cooking them as the citric acid breaks down the mushroom material. Find a detailed guide here: https://doubleblind-mag.com/mushrooms/how-to-take-shrooms/lemon-tek/

LSD: Lysergic acid diethylamide (LSD) is a classical hallucinogen that was first produced in 1938 from a chemical (lysergic acid) derived from ergot, a fungus that infects grain, by Swiss chemist Albert Hoffman. It is one of the most well-known psychedelic substances, used extensively in therapy in the 1960s – as well as by the hippie counter-culture. It is considered one of the "least harmful drugs" – second only to psilocybin. The active component of LSD interacts with serotonin receptors in the brain, just like psilocybin and DMT (the active component in Ayahuasca).

MACRODOSING: Consuming a large enough dose of a psychedelic medicine to have a hallucinogenic experience – the typically profound, classic psychedelic journey. A macrodose tends to result in drastic perceptual, cognitive, and emotional changes. A macrodose could be anywhere between a threshold dose – the dose at which perceptual changes just become noticeable – and a heroic dose, where one often has deep and intense effects – such as ego death/dissolution.

MAGIC MUSHROOMS: See *Psilocybin*.

MAPS: Founded in 1986, the Multidisciplinary Association for Psychedelic Studies (MAPS) is a nonprofit research and educational organization that develops medical, legal, and cultural contexts for people to benefit from the careful uses of psychedelics and cannabis. Founded by Rick Doblin, MAPS has raised more than $130 million for psychedelic research and education over the course of the past 35 years, leading the way in MDMA-assisted therapy research.

MAOI: Monoamine oxidase inhibitors (MAOIs) are an older type of antidepressant and anxiolytic medications (such as Marplan, Nardil, and Parnate) that have largely been phased out by newer drugs with fewer side effects, such as selective serotonin reuptake inhibitors (SSRIs). In nature, MAOIs are known to "activate" the DMT in Ayahuasca. Plants to avoid, unless you want a much more intense and longer journey, include Syrian rue; yohimbe (also known as quebrachine); and passionflower. MAOIs interact with numerous other prescription and over-the-counter drugs, including certain anesthetics, painkillers, migraine medications, sedatives, antihistamines, antidepressants, sleeping pills, and allergy meds.

MDMA: First synthesized by Merck in 1912 – from an oily liquid extracted from the sassafras tree's bark or fruit – producing 3,4-methylenedioxy-N-methylamphetamine. It produces a heart-opening, euphoric feeling (because it is an entactogen) that begins about 45 minutes after ingestion, and lasts 3-6 hours (unless you also consume a booster). Other benefits include increased energy levels, improved mood, sharper mental clarity, and reduced anxiety. Note: MDMA is not the same as the street drugs Ecstasy or Molly, both of which contain MDMA as the active agent but may also contain unknown – and sometimes dangerous – cutting agents or adulterants.

MEDITATION: A mind-body practice used by many people, often as part of integration practices with psychedelic medicine experiences. Meditation, which has been used for thousands of years, focuses on developing an intentional focus of thought – while blocking out the noise and random thoughts that often enter our minds – keeping focus on breathing. It can help us lower stress and blood pressure levels, help us be more connected to a higher power, and improve our abilities to focus.

MESCALINE: a naturally occurring, gentle, and heart-opening psychedelic protoalkaloid found in certain cacti (best known are the peyote and San Pedro/Huachuma), and known for its hallucinogenic effects, which are comparable to those of LSD and psilocybin. Mescaline became a "thing" when Aldous Huxley took the medicine for the first time in the 1950s and wrote a series of essays that was then published in book form with the title *The Doors of Perception*.

MICRODOSING: consuming a tiny fraction (5-10 percent) of a full dose of a psychedelic medicine, allowing many of the benefits of the medicine to be utilized without the hallucinogenic (psychedelic) experience. While research has been mostly anecdotal, we are seeing studies that suggests that microdosing can bring about some of the benefits observed with full-dose treatment without causing the intense and sometimes negative hallucinatory experiences. For others, microdosing is also used as a tool for gently "getting to know" a psychedelic medicine before deciding to complete a macrodose journey.

NEUROPLASTICITY: is the ability of neural networks in your brain to change through growth and reorganization – in response to life experiences – creating new neurons and building new networks. Old thinking had the brain cease growing/learning at the end of childhood. Emerging research suggests that there's a clear link between psychedelics and neuroplasticity, and that using psychedelics may help you make long-term, positive changes to your brain. Your brain actually has increased neural plasticity when consuming psychedelics, providing an opportunity to make significant changes to your life that may last a long time.

POST-TRAUMATIC STRESS: a disorder that develops in some people who have experienced a serious, deadly, shocking, scary, or dangerous event in which people's fight or flight response is extremely exaggerated, resulting in being triggered into extreme action from sometimes innocuous situations. PTS, or PTSD as it is often referred to, can happen to anyone in almost any situation. We mostly attribute PTSD to veterans and first responders, but anyone facing a traumatic situation can experience PTSD. Psychedelics seem to be a breakthrough protocol for reducing, eliminating PTS.

PSILOCYBIN: a naturally occurring psychedelic produced by more than 200 species of fungi, and which have been used for as many as 10,000 years – maybe even longer. Hallucinogenic mushrooms – so-called Magic Mushrooms – include species that contain psychedelic substances, including psilocybin; these mushrooms can be found across the globe: 53 are found in Mexico, 22 in the United States and Canada, 19 in Australia and the surrounding islands, 16 in Europe, 15 in Asia, and 4 in Africa… though new species are still being discovered.

PSYCHEDELIC: a mental state induced by certain compounds, and characterized by a profound sense of intensified sensory perception, sometimes accompanied by severe perceptual distortion and hallucinations and by extreme feelings of either euphoria… or despair. These medicines work by stimulating, suppressing, or modulating the activity of various neurotransmitters in the brain, which causes a temporary chemical imbalance in the brain, leading to hallucinations and other effects. The term psychedelic, first coined by British psychiatrist Humphrey Osmond, is composed of the Greek term *psyche (soul, spirit, mind)* and *dēlos (to manifest, to reveal)* … thus it translates into "soul manifesting" or "spirit revealing."

PSYCHONAUT: a label used to describe people who regularly seek out and take psychedelic journeys deep into their consciousness – usually at higher-than-average doses. Like the term psychedelic, the roots of psychonaut come from the Greek – with the prefix *psyche* meaning spirit, soul, or mind, while the suffix *naut* pertains to sailing; therefore, a common definition of a psychonaut is a "sailor of the soul." Less about healing and more about exploring and understanding, these people deliberately enter altered states of consciousness to explore the hidden depths of the human psyche.

PURGING: a term used in psychedelics that refers to the release of bad energy, bad memories, bad thoughts. It is the process of eliminating energy, emotions, and trauma from the body – whether via traditional bodily experiences (vomiting and defecation, especially with Ayahuasca) or other purging, such as laughing, yawning, chanting, crying, shaking, sweating, and hacking. Not all people purge – and most certainly people purge in different ways – and even in different ways depending on the medicine.

RAPÉ (SNUFF): also known as shamanic snuff, it is a specific type of tobacco used in some sacred ceremonies, and that is distinct from the type of tobacco that is found in cigarettes. And unlike cigarettes, this type of tobacco is not typically smoked. Instead, most people snuff the compound into their noses.

SET & SETTING: a phrase used to emphasize one of the key tenants related to the consumption of psychedelic medicine – and made famous in the early 1960s by Dr. Timothy Leary, a psychologist who spent his career advocating for the benefits of psychedelic drugs. Set describes the mental preparation one needs to do for a psychedelic experience; it deals with getting your mind in the right space – the right mindset for a healing journey. Setting deals with having a safe and comfortable place to experience a psychedelic journey. The more time you spend with getting set and setting correct, the less likely you will experience a challenging ("bad") trip.

SHADOW SELF: a term made popular by Swiss Psychoanalyst Carl Jung, in which he theorized that personality can be separated into 'that which we are conscious of – the ego – and elements 'that which we are unconscious of – the shadow self. Have you ever felt you have worn a mask or been like a chameleon to fit into certain situations? That's your shadow – and Jung believed that to have a more fulfilling life, the shadow must be integrated with the conscious… brought into the light. Psychedelic medicines have a way of stripping through all the layers and dark shadows and allowing us to see and address and heal our shadows. In most cases, that results in a reduction of ego, but in some cases, the ego can actually be greatly enhanced.

SSRI: a class of prescription drugs that are meant to work on making more serotonin available, but new research is questioning what actually causes depression – and that SSRIs are not the solution. Selective serotonin reuptake inhibitors (SSRIs) are typically used as antidepressants in the treatment of major depressive disorder, anxiety disorders, and other psychological conditions. SSRIs are one type of antidepressant; other types include tricyclic antidepressants (TCAs), serotonin and norepinephrine reuptake inhibitors (SNRIs), norepinephrine and dopamine reuptake inhibitors (NDRIs), monoamine oxidase inhibitors (MAO-Is) – all designed to relieve the symptoms of depression.

TRIPSITTER: sometimes known as a sober sitter, it is a term used in psychedelics to describe a person who remains sober to ensure the safety of the person taking a psychedelic journey – someone who sits with the person while they are under the influence the medicine. A tripsitter is with you both for harm reduction (to protect you), as well as for helping handle anything that might disrupt the setting (such as keeping the music going, getting drinks or snacks, answering the door/phone). *Compare to guide/facilitator.*

TRAUMA: a disturbing or hurtful event or experience that often results in pain, shame, guilt, fear, anger – especially if the trauma is not addressed. Trauma can come in many forms, from major traumas (such as physical and psychological abuses) to minor traumas (such as the withholding of love or safety). It's clear, even from the early research, that psychedelics can be an invaluable tool for healing all types of trauma, but especially deep psychological emotional traumas that have been suppressed for years. Recommended reading: Dr. Gabor Mate's *The Myth of Normal* and Dr. Paul Conti's *Trauma: The Invisible Epidemic*.

TREATMENT-RESISTANT DEPRESSION: a term used in clinical psychiatry to describe a condition where standard depression treatments are not enough; it refers to people with major depressive disorder who do not respond positively to a course of appropriate antidepressant medication and talk-therapy within a certain time. Symptoms can range from mild to severe and may require trying a number of approaches to identify what helps – including psychedelic medicines.

TRYPTAMINES: are a naturally occurring neurotransmitter in the brain that is derived from tryptophan and can be converted into other neurotransmitters, such as serotonin and melatonin. Tryptamine psychedelics – including LSD, psilocybin, and DMT – are also labeled as psychotomimetic, hallucinogenic, psychedelic, or entheogenic; they result in shifts in perception, ego-death, and introspection.

ACKNOWLEDGMENTS

THE IDEA: This book only exists because of three people; yes, I researched, interviewed, and wrote the physical words you just finished reading, but the bulk of the credit goes to my partner and wife, Jenny Hansen. The other person who deserves credit for the book is Jesse Gould.

Jenny is the love of my life, the best part of my life, and my adventure partner – in whichever ways the adventure of life takes us. She has been my go-to for everything psychedelic for the past several years, introducing me to many key experts and professionals in the field. She has graciously been my sounding board and editor. She is an integral part of this book; her personality is woven through out it.

Jesse is the founder of Heroic Hearts Project, one of the nonprofits that will be receiving funds from the sale of this book. Jenny heard Jesse on a podcast several years ago, and the rest is history. Jesse's story is well-known, thus not in the book. He is a decorated Army Ranger who came home suffering from the traumas of war. He self-medicated with alcohol, as many veterans (and first responders) do, and refused the pill-pushing from the VA in search of something that might cure him rather than simply mask the symptoms. Amazingly, he uncovered Ayahuasca in his research – and he went down to Peru to seek healing. That healing led to his mission of helping other veterans receive the healing he received.

THE CORE: This book only exists because of the generosity of 23 people, who were willing to open themselves up for you – so that you could understand their existence pre- and post-psychedelics. Some of these people were dealing with major traumas and really struggling, while others were soul-searching, seeking their truths, their true-selves. The people in this book are my heroes – for deciding to shout from the rooftop that they have been involved with intentional psychedelic experiences… for sharing their truths.

It may be hard to understand, but it is amazing to see more and more people bravely raising their hands and sharing their psychedelic experiences – including the traumas that had been holding them back from living their best lives. More amazing to me is that some of the people are bravely sharing at least some of their stories on LinkedIn and other social media.

THE BOOK: So many people to thank here. First, I have to thank some people that are not even included in the book, but who helped out behind the scenes, including Tammy Le, Donna Loeffler, and Dr. Rick Barnett. I also want to acknowledge the support from Sisters in Psychedelics, a unique platform for supporting women (and men) in psychedelics, and for the support of Empathic.Health.

I also have to give mega-thanks to two other authors who shared their expertise by offering their takes on macrodosing and microdosing. So, special thanks to Matt Zemon for writing the introduction to macrodosing – and who has a wonderful companion book to this one: *Psychedelics for Everyone*. Also grateful to C.J. Spotswood for writing the introduction to microdosing – and for recommending a few people with microdosing stories; C.J. also has a fantastic book: *The Microdosing Handbook*.

You would not be holding such a beautiful book if it were not for my wonderful designer, Michelle Fairbanks. And, again, I need to thank Jenny for her editing and proofing of this book prior to printing, as well as dear friend Kelli Dickerson in helping with editing and proofreading.

Finally, I have asked several key colleagues and friends to participate in various types of research relating to the format, title, and design of the book. Major thanks to Lea Bell, Ed Ashley, Brad Hansen, Julie Smarkos, and the one and only Robbie Nodine.

THE BLURBS/REVIEWS: A special place exists in my heart for the folks who took a chunk of time to read an advance copy of the book and share their thoughts, reactions, and reviews. Much gratitude to David Bronner, Tim Moore, Carlos Tanner, Floris Wolswijk, Douglas Finkelstein, Jesse Gould, Gaetano G.M. Lardieri, Dr. Andrea Pennington and Nicholas Levich.

THE RESULT: Thanks go to you, dear reader, for purchasing this book. Not only will you learn all you need to know about psychedelic medicines, but the money you spent purchasing this book will be going directly into the hands of several key nonprofits in this healing space, including: Heroic Hearts Project, Chacruna, and the Fireside Project.

In other words, by purchasing this book, you have an impact on saving multiple lives – your own and others seeking healing. Thank you... and bon voyage!

PRAISE

for Triumph Over Trauma

Dr. Randall Hansen does an incredible service for all of us, compiling amazing stories of people healing debilitating conditions and traumatic life experiences through intentional journeying with psychedelic medicines.

This book demystifies and destigmatizes this still all too often misunderstood and underappreciated modality of healing, that promises to help so many who are trapped in anguish and suffering.

I'm grateful that the power of these first-person accounts, along with Dr. Hansen's insightful writing, will help people feel comfortable accessing what in many cases can be literally lifesaving medicine.

–DAVID BRONNER, Cosmic Engagement Officer,
Dr. Bronner's Magic Soaps

By laying the foundation on the basics of psychedelic medicines, Triumph Over Trauma provides readers the opportunity to fully empathize with the personal, human stories shared in the case studies. In this way, the book stays true to form of what healing and transformational journeys consist of: knowledge gathering, preparation, experience, and integration.

I am confident that by the end of this book, you will feel a personal connection and gratitude toward at least one of the people who have shared their story. Any book that can elicit those feelings is a book worth reading.

–DOUG FINKELSTEIN, Chief Empathy Officer, *Empathic.Health*

I had the honor of being asked to read an advance copy of Dr. Hansen's book, *Triumph over Trauma*.

As a member of the psychedelic's industry (we supply naturally derived GMP psilocybin to researchers) I was keen to read it.

Dr. Hansen has delivered a wondered primer for those new to the exciting promise provided by psychedelics. He covers the history, misconceptions, misinformation and outright lies that have caused so many patients to have been deprived access these wonderful plant-based compounds. He underscores the urgent need for alternative treatments in a world facing multiple crises: "a mental health crisis; a suicide crisis; an addiction crisis; a spiritual crisis; a wellness crisis; an abuse crisis; a pill-popping crisis; a HEALING crisis."

Through the in-depth history lesson and the sharing of intimate stories from people with actual psychedelic experiences, the book provides a comprehensive look into how psychedelics can address these crises.

I have often said that as participants in psychedelic medicine, we are in the "industry of hope," hope for a normal life, able to look forward to living your life. It is my opinion that traditional treatment of mental health patients is too often focused on making them easier to life with, not making their lives better. Psychedelics offer the promise of a normal life.

I recommend this book whether you are new to psychedelics or if you have already been immersed in it.

–TIM MOORE, CEO, *Havn Life Sciences*

Dr. Randall Hansen beautifully leverages the power of stories to show how psychedelics can heal. He emphatically rejects the daily cocktail of pills and embraces the mind-expanding effects of psychedelics. In an ever more isolated world, Dr. Hansen offers a space for individual stories, with broadly applicable lessons.

– FLORIS WOLSWIJK, Founder of *Blossom*

Dr. Randall Hansen's book is exactly what modern society needs right now to guide our curiosity about psychedelics. The book provides a comprehensive collection of information about the various psychedelic medicines accessible to us, with their history, chemistry, research, and reports of profound healing.

As humankind becomes more aware that the pharmaceutical companies we used to look to for the solutions are simply not able to reach the root causes of our afflictions, Dr. Hansen's book demonstrates that in many cases psychedelics and psychedelic therapies are proving to be more effective than pharmaceutical medications.

No matter our race or heritage, our ancestors used psychedelic plant medicines for countless generations, and some cultures on Earth still do.

This book is a reminder to all of us that our ancestral wisdom of psychedelic medicines was not primitive or inferior. If we want to restore harmony to our health, our communities, and our environment, the use of psychedelics may be the greatest step forward to achieving those goals.

I'm so glad to know this book will accelerate the safe and beneficial use of psychedelics, and in turn accelerate the paradigm shift that is so direly needed in the world.

–**CARLOS TANNER,** Director, *Ayahuasca Foundation*

In addition to providing the necessary base level education, this book presents an intimate look into the personal stories of transformation that accompany intentional psychedelic use. It's rare to get such an honest and open look into what the personal healing process actually looks like. And Dr. Randall S. Hansen has managed to do this in such a way where the stories aren't embellished or sensationalized. In fact, seeing the pain, the struggle, and the triumph is part of what makes this body of work so compelling. This is a must-read for anyone considering a psychedelic journey of their own!

–**NICHOLAS LEVICH,** Co-Founder,
Psychedelic Passage

Dr. Hansen has compiled a compelling group of real-life stories of people who experienced healing through the use of psychedelics. For those who are psychedelic-curious or wanting to prepare for an upcoming ceremony, Triumph over Trauma can help demystify the sacred medicines, and give you a glimpse into the types of experiences that await. Also included is a list of frequently asked questions and basic info on a variety of substances that make this a practical and useful exploration into the healing potential of psychedelics.

–**DR. ANDREA PENNINGTON,** Integrative Psychedelic Physician

After decades of being buried, psychedelics are once again sprouting in the Western world and changing our views on mental health, nature, and community. This rediscovery is already bringing in a new era of research and understanding but, more importantly, will provide millions with new ways to heal and thrive. In his book, *Triumph Over Trauma*, Dr. Randall Hansen explores the history as well as the future implications of psychedelics in the Western world.

Dr. Randall Hansen curates an expansive set of content to tell the reader exactly why this is a really big deal for each of us and our society at large. The first-person accounts also bring the book home and make it unique. At the end of the day, this is about people and how we all deserve the right to heal from our trauma and expand our self-understanding. Whether you are a person just entering space or have been working with psychedelics for years, this book has something for everyone.

Now is a time to celebrate these substances and share our personal stories. Now is the time to bring in a new era of mental healing and community. Our veterans need access to these medicines now. Our society needs access to these medicines now.

–JESSE GOULD, Former Army Ranger, Founder, and President of *Heroic Hearts Project*

Dr. Randall Hansen has provided us with the right book, at the right time, for all the right reasons. Triumph Over Trauma will provide you with empowering personal stories and journeys that will educate and empower you about Entheogenic Medicines. Americans and Humanity are going through a turbulent and interesting paradigm shift these days coming out of a global pandemic and dynamic paradoxical political climates which have separated us. The plant medicines are working to bring us all back together as one. They are breaking through on a grand global scale even beyond our planet as research is being conducted on how plants are going to survive in space. Triumph Over Trauma is the right set and setting at the moment.

–GAETANO G.M. LARDIERI, Global Researcher and Transhumanist

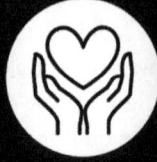

FACILITATOR TIP

One of the best ways to expand your connections and knowledge of psychedelics is by joining your local Psychedelic Society, many of which are managed on Meetup. These organizations have casual meetings, integration circles, speakers, and more – usually a combination of in-person and electronic meetings.

INSPIRING QUOTE

"With psychedelics... there is this epiphany that everything is connected. That we're all tiny little beings on a huge planet. If you pull back and see the big picture, you see that we are all one organism, interconnected or interdependent."

– DR. JULIE HOLLAND, M.D.

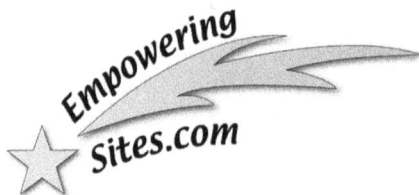

www.ingramcontent.com/pod-product-compliance
Lightning Source LLC
Chambersburg PA
CBHW062119020426
42335CB00013B/1030